The Foundations of Primary Care (OWL

DARING TO BE DIFFERENT

The Foundations of Primary Care

DARING TO BE DIFFERENT

JOACHIM P STURMBERG
MBBS DRACOG MFamMed FRACGP PhD

A/Prof of General Practice
Monash University, Melbourne, Australia
Conjoint A/Prof of General Practice
Newcastle University, Newcastle, Australia

With a contribution by
CARMEL M MARTIN

Foreword by
IAN R MCWHINNEY

Radcliffe Publishing
Oxford • Seattle

Radcliffe Publishing Ltd
18 Marcham Road
Abingdon
Oxon OX14 1AA
United Kingdom

www.radcliffe-oxford.com
Electronic catalogue and worldwide online ordering facility.

British Library Cataloguing in Publication Data

A catalogue record for this book is available from the British Library.

ISBN-10 1 84619 081 9
ISBN-13 978 1 84619 081 0

Typeset by Egan Reid Ltd, Auckland, New Zealand
Printed and bound by Alden (Malaysia)

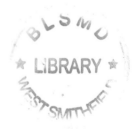

To my wife Birgit and children Björn,
Catrina, Kristian and René

Contents

Foreword

Medicine has a long history. For years, thinkers in family medicine and psychiatry have worked to change the clinical method that has dominated medicine since the 19th century. One outcome has been the patient-centred clinical method. The essence of this method is that the doctor's task is not finished unless he or she has ascertained the meaning of the illness for the patient.

How modern that sounds! Yet how old it is. Before the 19th century, many physicians diagnosed patients, not diseases. The advances in medicine in the 19th and 20th centuries gradually changed the idea of diagnosis to diagnosis of a disease. In 1926, Crookshank remarked that the new textbooks on diagnosis 'gave excellent schemes for the physical examination of the patient, whilst strangely ignoring, almost completely, the psychical (sic)'.[1] Indeed these controversies about diagnosis have been going on since the time of the ancient Greeks, when the Cnidians classified the patient's illness in accordance with a taxonomy of diseases and the Coans did not separate the disease from the person. The best physicians have always tried to find the balance between the two ideas. When seen in historical perspective, the patient-centred clinical method has restored the balance which had become too much askew.

I mention this example to illustrate the importance of seeing medicine in its historical perspective and of being curious about where our ideas come from. The more we can trace these ideas to their origins, the less likely are we to make wrong decisions.

Joachim Sturmberg has written an important book, which I sincerely hope the reformers of our healthcare system will study carefully. It is also a riveting read, including Carmel Martin's contribution to the two chapters at the end. With great erudition and strong arguments, Sturmberg lays out a plan that leads to a goal to which we all aspire – a healthcare system based on primary care and primary health care that expresses the historic values of medicine and adapts itself to the complexity of modern medicine.

The ideas of primary care and primary health care were introduced almost 100 years ago by the Dawson Report, in the UK.[2] One cannot read this report now without being impressed by its wisdom. It has stood the test of time, and the evidence for its effectiveness is overwhelming.[3] So is the evidence for the relationship between doctor and patient as the most effective and efficient way of providing care. It is crucial that the relationship be unconditional: the family physician must never say, for example, 'This is not my field'. Patients must be assured that any problem they have will be attended to. Referral to another physician may be necessary, but does not mean the end of the relationship.

So important is this relationship that we must resist attempts to divide it. Once it ceases to be unconditional, there is no end to the fragmentation that may ensue. None of us can be present for our patients all the time, day in day out, especially in the fast and fevered pace of our modern lives. We should not expect ourselves to be perfect, but do our utmost to nurture the relationship.

Rather than replenishing the family physician workforce, governments have stated their intention to substitute nurse practitioners for family physicians. The nurse–doctor relationship is extremely important and has the potential for improving health and health care. When doctor and nurse are working closely together with a patient, there will be overlap, which they will work out together and which the patient will be accustomed to. But substitution is going too far. The core skill of medicine is clinical diagnosis and therapy. Physicians spend four or more years learning these skills. Nursing also has core skills, different from medicine, but just as important. When brought together in harmony, these two sets of skills improve patient care and enable doctors and nurses to learn from each other. I am afraid that substituting nurses for doctors in the role of clinical diagnosis will have several consequences. First, it will blur the skill sets between two distinct professions. Second, according to Sturmberg, costs will probably increase. Third, and most worrying, it could compromise care, reducing the opportunities for physicians to know their patients and limiting the establishment of a doctor–patient relationship. So often, the first and last words a patient speaks holds the key to a problem, and what appears to be a minor illness can become very complex.

It is time for some hard thinking about teamwork. Without it, we may find that we have created a monster. The majority of patients attending family physicians can be diagnosed and treated by the physician alone. One of the most effective teams is the doctor–nurse duo working together with the same patients. These work together day in and day out in a relationship that has a long history. Another well-tried team is a nurse working as a liaison between a patient and other nurses or physicians. An example is a nurse who assesses patients having acute care in the home, and reports to the patient's physician.

The doctor–nurse team may be enhanced by other members for particular patients, for instance a social worker. Once the team is enhanced, it is important that it meets together periodically. Another team is the one assembled for one particular patient, such as a physician, dietician, social worker and clinical psychologist for a patient with an eating disorder.

Patients with multiple morbidities have many different needs. Much can be done for them if their needs can be properly assigned. The number of patients with these needs is growing as more people enter the 90 plus age bracket, and children with Down's syndrome and other disorders grow into adulthood. The organisation of a large and multifarious team is a difficult task. Good communication is paramount, and responsibility for all decisions should be clearly assigned. Any member of the team may be its leader, and all should be skilled in team leadership. The key to good teamwork is to devote time to the needs of the team members as well as the patients. The cautionary words about teamwork in the book are a must read for anyone who has the interests of primary care at heart.

As I read this book, I found myself examining some of the beliefs that drive the career decisions of physicians and other health professionals. For example, the belief in the 'explosion of knowledge' convinces physicians that they will have to divide their knowledge into smaller and small segments, leading to more and more specialties – a process that seems to be unravelling the healthcare system. Knowledge was said to be exploding in the 1950s and 1960s when I started in practice. In fact the opposite is the case. The advance of science simplifies knowledge. One discovery can change an unruly mass of data into a single knowledge-driven act. The discovery of the Wasserman test, for example, cleared away years of supposition and gave us one simple procedure for diagnosing syphilis. The discovery of insulin did the same for diabetes. Nearer to our time, in the 1950s, what we now call polymyalgia rheumatica was separated from rheumatoid arthritis, and steroid treatment gave patients instant relief.

When I began practising in London, Ontario in the 1960s, there were at least six general internists who were in constant demand for their wide experience of medicine. Now, the general internist has almost disappeared from our hospitals. More and more, family physicians are stepping into the breach. But, in many urban jurisdictions, family physicians have deserted the hospitals and have given up home care, which until recently kept them in touch with complex illnesses.

A recent trend among some general practitioners is to tell their patients that only one problem will be attended to at each visit. We soon learn in family practice that patients often present more than one problem and that their main problem may be presented last. There are reasons for this. The problem may be a source of shame, and the patient may fear censure or ridicule; or the problem may have dire consequences and it may take courage to mention it. We should always bear in mind that the presenting complaint may not be the whole story, so that we give time and space for patients to express what is on their minds. A patient in anguish, or bereaved, or in despair, already has more than one problem.

Does the refusal to deal with more than one problem in a single visit signal the end of compassion in medicine? Continuity of care, comprehensiveness of practice, and commitment to patients over long periods of time are so essential to family practice that it is difficult to see how it can survive without them.

Ian R McWhinney OC MD
Emeritus Professor of Family Medicine
The University of Western Ontario
Schulich School of Medicine and Dentistry
Centre for Studies in Family Medicine
November 2006

REFERENCES

1 Crookshank F. The theory of diagnosis, part one. *Lancet.* 1926; **November 6**: 939–42.

2 Starfield B, Shi L and Macinko J. Contribution of primary care to health systems and health. *Milbank Quarterly.* 2005; **83**: 457–502.

3 Lord Dawson. *Interim Report on the Future Provisions of Medical and Allied Services.* London: United Kingdom Ministry of Health. Consultative Council on Medical Allied Services. HMSO, 1920.

Acknowlegements

Over the past 20 years many friends and colleagues have subtly and mostly unknowingly contributed to this book. In particular I am most grateful to Ian McWhinney, Michael Balint, Alvan Feinstein, Hannes Pauli and Barbara Starfield, who through their writings sensitised and confronted me to reflect on my views and my work as a clinician, and who led me to explore medicine and general practice from an academic perspective.

However without the many reflective conversations between consultations, during teaching sessions, in meetings and over conference dinners, the book would never have eventuated. It is with great pleasure to especially acknowledge (in alphabetical order) Lyn Clearihan, George Freeman, Per Fugelli, Daniel Lam, Carmel Martin, Stewart Mennin, Mark Moes, Leon Piterman, Dimity Pond and Sandy Reid for generously sharing their insights about medicine in general and general practice in particular.

Then again without a catalyst writing would not have started. I thank Gillian Nineham from Radcliffe Publishing for her inspiring Quebec lecture and her subsequent support in the project.

Writing helps to clarify one's thoughts, but clarity requires comment from outside. For their critical review of the manuscript I am particularly indebted to (in alphabetical order) Liz Farmer, Richard Oak and Dimity Pond.

I gratefully acknowledge Michael Klein who kindly agreed to share a couple of his most memorable healing stories.

And finally I am most appreciative to Ian McWhinney for kindly agreeing to write the foreword for the book.

Copyright permissions

Fig 8.1   Copyright Marshall Clemens, by permission of idiagram (www.idiagram.com)

Fig 10.1   Reprinted from: New England Journal of Medicine, 344(26), Green L, Fryer G, Yawn B, Lanier D, Dovey S, The Ecology of Medical Care Revisited, 2021–2025, Copyright 2001, with permission from Massachusetts Medical Society

Fig 10.2   Reprinted from: New England Journal of Medicine, 344(26), Green L, Fryer G, Yawn B, Lanier D, Dovey S, The Ecology of Medical Care Revisited, 2021–2025, Copyright 2001, with permission from Massachusetts Medical Society

Fig 11.1   Reprinted from: Ethical dilemmas arising from implementation of the European guidelines on cardiovascular disease prevention in clinical practice. A descriptive epidemiological study. Getz L, Kirkengen A, Hetlevik I, Romundstad S, Sigurdsson. Scandinavian Journal of Primary Health Care, www.tandf.no/primhealth, 2004; 22(4): 2002–2008, with permission from Taylor & Francis AS

Fig 11.2   Reprinted from: Engel G. The Clinical Application of the Biopsychosocial Model. American Journal of Psychiatry 1980; 137(5): 535–544, with permission from American Psychiatric Association

Fig 12.2   Reprinted from: From science to everyday clinical practice. Need for systematic evaluation of research findings. Lauritzen T, Mainz J, Lassen J. Scandinavian Journal of Primary Health Care, www.tandf.no/primhealth, 1999; 17(1): 6–10, with permission from Taylor & Francis AS

Fig 16.1   Reprinted from: Lancet, Vol 360(9346), Poulton R, Caspi A, Milne BJ, Thomson WM, Taylor A, Sears MR, et al. Association between children's experience of socioeconomic disadvantage and adult health: a life-course study, 1640–1645, Copyright 2002, with permission from Elsevier

Tab 16.1   Reprinted from: Social Science and Medicine, Vol 36(8), Lundberg O. The Impact of Childhood Living Conditions on Illness and Mortality in Adulthood, 1047–1052, Copyright 1993, with permission from Elsevier

Introduction

We must be the change we wish to see in the world.

Gandhi

Medicine has a long and fine tradition. Humanistic values are the foundation of the healing profession, a point partly lost since scientific and technological advances gave rise to the promise of curing all disease in the late 19th century.

At the beginning of the 21st century, medicine worldwide is in a deep crisis – patients increasingly express their dissatisfaction with their medical care, and doctors feeling a loss of respect and standing in the community. In the western world the cry for evidence and a hostile medico-legal environment have perpetuated the demise of *the magic of healing* for the rise of *the commercial relationship of buying and selling perfect health*.

The media has successfully contributed to the widespread illusion that health care always achieves perfect results, even in the most dire circumstances. It is not surprising that these expectations have placed enormous pressures on the healthcare system to provide the necessary resources to achieve these largely unrealistic goals. For governments, health has become a bottomless pit fuelled by self-indulgence of doctors and patients alike.

Whether we like it or not, this is the world in which we live and work, a world of great contradictions, a world that nevertheless, when feeling ill, puts its faith in doctors, and a world that still entrusts us to discharge our obligations and responsibilities when needed.

Medicine remains as exciting as ever. Albert Einstein once said 'The world will not evolve past its current state of crisis by using the same thinking that created the situation'.

The history and philosophy of medicine provide the foundations to understanding the 'current crisis' and complexity, and systems thinking may provide the foundations to moving beyond it.

INTRODUCTION

The Foundations of Primary Care aims to paint a contemporary picture of medicine rooted in its historical and philosophical traditions. The picture is painted in five sections, all interconnected and merging into one through the metaphor of the healthcare vortex. Each picture covers one aspect of health and health care – its history and philosophy, its various practices and its social engagement in society, and its emergence as a dynamically responsive discipline focused on the improvement of personal health.

The Foundations of Primary Care aims to provide an overview and a synthesis of the matters that have shaped medical thinking and medical practice and that remain essential for the emerging health system of the 21st century. This book aims to provide contextual perspectives on medical care, thus having to limit itself succinctly to pertinent issues. Readers who want to further their interest in particular issues are provided with a selected 'Further reading' list.

It is my hope that readers gain an understanding of the complex interconnected nature of health, illness and disease, and their relationships to medical care. Health and health care are a complex adaptive system – metaphorically described through the healthcare vortex. Complex adaptive systems are governed by their core value, and their behaviour is based on the repeated application of a few simple rules.

The Foundations of Primary Care makes the case that the core value of medical care is the improvement of *personal health*, the value inherent and constant since the beginnings of medicine, and that the achievement of *personal health* depends on an *ongoing personal healing relationship with the doctor.*

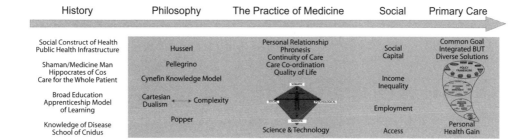

SECTION ONE

Historical perspective of medicine: from shaman to modern physician

Medicine . . . is a human creation cradled in the primate programme.

Tiger and Fox [1]

Any system is grounded in its own history – the past lives on in the present. Gaining a historical perspective on medicine is a very useful way of achieving a greater depth of understanding of medicine and, in particular, primary health care at the beginning of the 21st century. This section of the book traces the thought and achievements of the leading thinkers, researchers and educators and their contribution to the growth of our discipline.

History shows us how changes in thinking can lead to the revision of conventional wisdom. It explains the impact these changes have on the discipline and on society at large. History also teaches us that at times changes may turn full circle – nowhere is this more obvious than in the return to a holistic model of health and health care and the rejection of the pure biomedical (man–machine) model of disease based on Descartes' mind–body split.

Chapter 1 will give a brief outline of the historical origins of our healing profession. Care for the sick and injured helped to secure the survival of the small group in hunter and gatherer societies. Medicine is both a social and a scientific construct.

As a social act medicine developed its specific rituals, which in turn shaped societal expectation relating to health and health care. The Romans translated the knowledge of environmental factors on the health and wellbeing of the population into the development of a sophisticated public health system.

Chapter 2 traces some of the 'milestones of medicine' in anatomy and physiology, population health, diagnostic technologies and therapeutics, all of which have given us the ability to successfully treat specific disease entities (as opposed to illness).

In Chapter 3 the influence of medical education on shaping medical frameworks and practices cannot be underestimated. Historically, medical training aimed to achieve 'educated men' over and above providing them with specific technical skills. A good education was seen as transcending subject matter, it was regarded as important to open the student's mind to the interconnected nature of man's life experiences. The education process made him a *doctor* – doctor meaning the learned one.

The fourth chapter outlines the long, and at times bitter, struggle of primary care to find its own identity and acceptance within the medical profession. The successes of the patient-centred approach and the desire to treat patients outside hospitals have greatly enhanced the status and the standing of the general practitioner/family physician in society.

The general practitioner/family physician is firmly embedded in the fabric of the community, understanding the individual as well as the larger societal aspects impacting on the health of the community. Greater understanding of disease mechanisms and treatment options has provided effective modalities to treat specific diseases; however the traditional approaches of 'talk, ritual and handing out medicines' have not changed, and remain the basis of effective health care.

CHAPTER 1

The history of medicine

THE ORIGINS OF MEDICINE: THE SHAMAN/MEDICINE MAN

To fully appreciate the 'role of the doctor' it is worth going back to the very origin of civilisation. Hunter and gatherer societies started to stay with and care for the sick and weak group members. Looking after group members was driven both by self-interest – loss of a member jeopardised the chances of survival of the group – and the perhaps rising awareness of one's own mortality. At that time all members of the group participated in the caring activities.

Caring for the sick became more sophisticated with the passing of time, and the first medical professional was born – the shaman or medicine man. The role of the shaman/medicine man combined three functions: curing the sick, directing communal sacrifice and escorting the dead to another world – today these roles are conducted by three different professions: the doctor, the priest and the undertaker.[2]

Though these functions have been separated in modern society they are still very much functions expected by our patients, and in fact play an important role in 'healing' the patient. Indeed the origin of the word 'medicine' refers to 'any object or practice regarded by primitive people as of magical efficacy'.[3]

THE SOCIAL NATURE OF MEDICINE

Medicine in these early days had an important social function – restoring the health of the sick enabled them to once again become fully functioning members of the group. The group's recognition of the importance of the shaman/medicine man for their survival granted him (the shaman/medicine man was almost always male) the privilege of not having to hunt. He was fed and often received gifts. Thus health and illness were constructed from a social perspective.[4,5]

THE NATURE OF ILLNESS

In the mythology of the shaman/medicine man illness was believed to be caused by the loss of 'animus' (Latin: soul, character, disposition), and that healing would be achieved by restoring this positive quality of health.[6] Another explanation attributes illness to the invasion of destructive external forces, and thus healing could only be achieved by fighting off of the demon.[2] Both explanations ascribe a symbolic property to the nature and experience of illness, a point explored in more detail in Chapter 11.

HEALING: THE SHAMAN'S/MEDICINE MAN'S WAY

People in early societies attributed their diseases and illnesses to the work of witches and sorcerers (assigning meaning/understanding the symbolism of their ailment), and believed that the medicine man, through his magical powers, would be able to extract these from their body.

Shamen/medicine men underwent rigorous initiation to gain their 'supernormal' powers, while others were basically learned experts (now called medical graduates). Their training made them knowledgeable in the magic potencies of various substances (now called medicines), and gave them the ritual skills of administering these.

Shamen commonly carried a variety of objects, such as feathers of valued birds, specially shaped stones or hallucinogenic plants, which all symbolised their magical powers in the healing process (not unlike today's 'white coat' and the stethoscope or X-ray machine).

THE SHAMAN/MEDICINE MAN HAS NOT DIED

The work and the success of a shaman depend as much on his magic as on his patients' beliefs. A successful shaman, and for that matter a successful doctor, understands his community and his patients' circumstances and expectations. The following story, kindly provided by Michael C Klein – Emeritus Professor of Family Practice and Pediatrics at the University of British Columbia, Canada, illustrates how 'shamanic traits' can at times be spectacularly successful.

THE GENERAL PRACTITIONER AS SHAMAN

In the early 1970s, Montreal was experiencing a wave of immigration of Jews from Arab countries. Having left their countries, fearing for their lives and livelihood, the new immigrants presented to general practitioners (GPs) with a range of psychosomatic illnesses. Mrs A's chief complaint delivered in French was: 'I swallowed my tonsils'. She was convinced that she had done so and was, based on my/our experience with other anxiety related displacements, not going to be easily disabused of this formulation. My prior negative experiences with working through a psychological formularisation of such severe somatisation in an unsophisticated patient, led me to a radical intervention.

I went upstairs to discuss the case with my friendly ear, nose and throat (ENT) surgeon. I requested that he engage with me in a little shamanism, requesting that he see the patient with me in his office. I requested that he put on his best and biggest head mirror, anesthetise the patient's throat and, with much fanfare, reach deep in her throat with the longest ring forceps he could find and announce that he had retrieved her tonsils and cured her. This he did as requested with dramatic effect: instant expressions of gratitude from the patient, whose symptoms disappeared immediately. The patient and her family remained in my practice for many years, and while other adaptation issues persisted for about 3–5 years in various family members, no symptoms of globus hystericus returned.

The family were shopkeepers in their country of origin. The man of the house had many employees, the woman many servants. On arrival in Montreal, the husband was unemployed, depressed and did not make a successful integration for many years. Meanwhile the wife was forced into a new and stressful role as head of the household, working outside the home for the first time. This pattern was well recognised and regularly associated with somatisation.

In my perhaps extreme intervention, I had decided that Western normative attempts to develop the psyche–soma insight, was not going to work. Moreover, it tended in my experience to lead to fixation of symptoms and chronic psychological problems: hence my radical and unorthodox treatment. Fortunately it worked. Neither I nor my ENT consultant lost our licenses, but it was risky business. And I did not engage in such theatrics again. I guess I will leave my rattles and masks at home.

As the next story shows, experienced and successful shamen are well attuned to medical developments, and are by no means averse to integrating these into their traditional treatments.

A SHAMAN–MEDICAL STUDENT COLLABORATION
When I was a second year medical student at Stanford circa 1962 I found myself on a six-month stint in Chiapus Mexico near Guatemala on a medical-anthropological project studying hypertension along the Pan American Highway. We thought that communities near the Highway would be under the strain of acculturation to Western values and would show more hypertension than those further removed from the Highway. It did not take long to determine that nobody had hypertension so there was nothing to study.

Meanwhile a typhoid epidemic hit my village of Aguacatenango and nearby villages, and people started getting very sick and were dying. Vincente, the infermero (nurse-dresser) assigned to the village got typhoid, and the Indian agency had no replacement. As one of his last acts before being taken out of the village, Vincente gave me the keys to the dispensary and showed me where the chloramphenicol (all we had at the time) was stored. So this medical student started to play doctor (or nurse). I had a little lab but it was not difficult to determine who had the disease, and I began dispensing the wonder drug. Most of my patients did well.

The village had four shamen called curanderos, three relatively young ones and one who must have been about 80 years old. The patients of the curanderos were not doing so well and deaths among their clientele were apparent to the villagers, who began to appear at the clinic of the hotshot medical student, much to the dismay of the younger curanderos, who became a bit threatened and threatening.

I had learned that diseases that we might classify as being in the realm of internal medicine were thought to be due to loss of soul. One cause was the evil eye (susto). Other causes of loss of soul were a fright or a chill from a cold wind or other natural phenomenon. Those due to susto required finding the 'witch' and killing her/him while the other causes would involve a curing ceremony designed to recapture the lost soul.

One afternoon the older curandero appeared at the clinic and asked for a private consultation. He explained to me that he had become acquainted with the use of chloroquine in the treatment of malaria and had been incorporating chloroquine into his curing ceremonies to good effect. He was not pleased with his results in the current epidemic.

I gave him a good supply of chloramphenicol. His patients did a little better than mine.

HIGHLIGHTS FROM EARLY MEDICAL PRACTICE

Societal perceptions and behaviours as well as the physician's role are deeply rooted in the history of medical care. Self-care and folk medicine co-existed with the care by doctors. The close link between medicine and religion reflects the symbolic nature of illness, thus studying religion and medicine concomitantly was a prerequisite for becoming a well-educated physician up to the early 19th century.

BABYLONIAN MEDICINE
Babylonian medicine and religion were closely interrelated, and medical practice was highly state regulated. Drugs were mostly derived from plants and were largely ineffective. Technical treatments included the dilatation of gonorrhoeal strictures with catheterisation.[7]

Medical practice of medicine was highly codified and state regulated. The Hammurabi Code (approximately 2000 BC), 'printed' on a black diorite block 8 feet tall,[8] reveals not only the practice, but also the fee entitlements of the doctor and his penalties for malpractice:

§ 215. If a doctor has treated a gentleman for a severe wound with a bronze lances and has cured the man, or has opened an abscess of the eye for a gentleman with the bronze lances and has cured the eye of the gentleman, he shall take ten shekels of silver.

§ 218. If the doctor has treated a gentleman for a severe wound with a lances of bronze and has caused the gentleman to die, or has opened an abscess of the eye for a gentleman and has caused the loss of the gentleman's eye, one shall cut off his hands.

§ 219. If a doctor has treated the severe wound of a slave of a poor man with a bronze lances and has caused his death, he shall render slave for slave.

§220. If he has opened his abscess with a bronze lances and has made him lose his eye, he shall pay money, half his price.

§ 221. If a doctor has cured the shattered limb of a gentleman, or has cured the diseased bowel, the patient shall give five shekels of silver to the doctor.

§ 224. If a cow doctor or a sheep doctor has treated a cow or a sheep for a severe wound and cured it, the owner of the cow or sheep shall give one-sixth of a shekel of silver to the doctor as his fee.

EGYPTIAN MEDICINE

As the Ebers and Smith papyri reveal, Egyptian medicine also had a strong link with religion. The concepts of disease included ideas of spirits, worms and intestinal decay. The Egyptians discovered and understood many diseases, and treatments included surgical procedures and cautery, and a wide variety of plant-based drugs. Copper salts, wine and frankincense were used as antiseptics.[7]

However when there was no identifiable reasons for disease, doctors and priests alike attributed them to spirits, and accordingly treated them with spells and magical potions:

> These words are to be spoken over the sick person. 'O Spirit, male or female, who lurks hidden in my flesh and in my limbs, get out of my flesh. Get out of my limbs!' This was a remedy for a mother and child.
>
> Come! You who drives out evil things from my stomach and my limbs. He who drinks this shall be cured just as the gods above were cured.
>
> This was added at the end of this cure: 'This spell is really excellent – successful many times.' It was meant to be said when drinking a remedy.[9]

GREEK MEDICINE

Not all patients in ancient Greece turned to physicians when ill, many turned to the Gods, like Asclepios (Roman spelling: Aesculapius) from the 6th century BC onwards. Asclepeias, temple-like buildings solely run by priests, sprang up everywhere to treat those in poor health. People came to bathe, sleep and meditate, often opioid induced, as it was believed that during sleep they were visited by Asclepios and his two daughters, Panacea and Hygeia. Snakes would crawl over them during the night and patients would wake in the morning cured.[7,9]

Hippocrates of Cos (460–380 BC) started to look at poor health and disease, using reasoning and observation, rather than attributing these to supernatural causes.

> Men believe only that it is a divine disease because of their ignorance and amazement.[9]

He introduced the concept of observation to medicine, developed theories of illnesses, and described the natural history of many diseases. His theory of the four humours influenced medical thinking well into the 18th century.

> He would observe thus in acute diseases; first, the countenance of the patient, if it be like those of persons in health, and more so, if like itself, for this is the best of all; whereas the most opposite to it is the worst, such as the following: a sharp nose, hollow eyes, collapsed temples; the ears cold, contracted, and their lobes turned out; the skin about the forehead

being rough, distended, and parched; the color of the whole face being green, black, livid, or leadcolored. If the countenance be such at the commencement of the disease, and if this cannot be accounted for from the other symptoms, inquiry must be made whether the patient has long wanted sleep; whether his bowels have been very loose; and whether he has suffered from want of food; and if any of these causes be confessed to, the danger is to be reckoned so far less; and it becomes obvious, in the course of a day and a night, whether or not the appearance of the countenance proceeded from these causes. But if none of these be said to exist, and if the symptoms do not subside in the aforesaid time, it is to be known that certain death is at hand.[7]

He also introduced the concept of prognosis and attempted to tell patients and relatives what was most likely to happen.[7]

I believe that it is an excellent thing for a physician to practice forecasting. He will carry out the treatment best if he knows beforehand from the present symptoms what will take place later.[9]

Thus a man will be the more esteemed to be a good physician, for he will be the better able to treat those aright who can be saved, from having anticipated everything; and by seeing and announcing beforehand those who will live and those who will die, he will thus escape censure.[7]

Not only is Hippocrates known for his holistic approach to medical practice and his belief in a diagnosing the patient, he provided ethical guidance to all doctors codified in the Hippocratic Oath.

Hippocrates was rivalled by the School of Cnidus which, through a reductionist conception (revitalised in the 20th century), emphasised to its students the necessity to diagnose the disease. Ultimately their lack of evidence led to its demise, whereas the Hippocratic School of Cos succeeded into our days.

ROMAN MEDICINE

Medicine in early Roman times had three domains, remedies being prescribed by the head of the family (pater familias), the Etruscan-based state religion, and the private medical practitioner educated in the Greek tradition.

Unwashed wool supplies very many remedies . . . it is applied . . . with honey to old sores. Wounds it heals if dipped in wine or vinegar . . . yolks of eggs . . . are taken for dysentery with the ash of their shells, poppy juice and wine. It is recommended to bathe the eyes with a decoction of the liver and to apply the marrow to those that are painful or swollen.[9]

During the 2nd century AD, Artaeus of Cappadocia described many diseases including diabetes, pneumonia, pleurisy, tuberculosis, tetanus, diphtheria and paralysis. His description of diabetes is remarkably accurate:

Diabetes is a wonderful affection, not very frequent among men, being a melting down of the flesh and limbs into urine. Its cause is of a cold and humid nature, as in dropsy. The course is the common one, namely, the kidneys and the bladder; for the patients never stop making water, but the flow is incessant, as if from the opening of aqueducts. The nature of the disease, then, is chronic, and it takes a long period to form; but the patient is short-lived, if the constitution of the disease be completely established; for the melting is rapid, the death speedy. Moreover, life is disgusting and painful; thirst unquenchable; excessive drinking, which, however, is disproportionate to the large quantity of urine, for more urine is passed; and one cannot stop them either from drinking or making water.[7]

Two of the outstanding Roman physicians were Cornelius Celsus (25 BC to 40 AD), who described the classical signs of inflammation – calor, rubor, tumour and dolour, and Galen of Pergamum (131–200 AD) whose influence lasted for almost 1500 years. He arguably was the most influential physician of all times. A prolific researcher of anatomy and physiology, and a highly respected clinician, he placed great emphasis on clinical history taking and examination. He was a proponent of the doctrine of humours first introduced by Hippocrates, and further sophisticated it.

The basic principle of life was a spirit (pneuma) drawn from the general World-spirit in the act of breathing. It encountered the body through the windpipe (trachea) and so passed to the lung and thence, through the arteria venalis (our pulmonary vein) to the left ventricle, where it encountered the blood. The food-substance from the intestines was carried as chyle by the portal vein to the liver. There it was converted into blood and endowed with a particular pneuma, the natural spirit, which bestowed the power of growth and nutrition. This venous blood then entered the vena cava, from which it passed upwards and downwards to the tissues of the body. A portion of this venous blood entered the right ventricle of the heart, from which most of it passed by way of the vena arterialis (our pulmonary artery) and its valve to the lungs for their nutrition. The small remaining part of the blood in the right ventricle passed by way of invisible pores in the interventricular septum into the left ventricle. There it mixed with the air, drawn in through the pulmonary vein, to produce arterial blood, which was there charged with a second type of pneuma, the vital spirit. Blood containing this pneuma passed into the arteries, endowing the various organs with activity. Such arterial blood as reached the brain became there charged with the third and noblest pneuma, the animal spirit, which passed through the hollow nerves to initiate motion and sensation in the organism. But the active mingling of the blood and the vital spirit in the left ventricle gave rise to injurious vapours. The vital spirit passed with the blood from the left ventricle into the arteries. The mitral valve, having only two cusps, was always slightly incompetent; so that blood mixed with vital spirit and injurious vapours passed back into the pulmonary vein and the lungs, by which the vapours were exhaled.[7]

Besides diet, massage and exercise, Galen's treatments included bleeding, purging, cupping and blistering.

Pedanius Dioscorides (circa 40–90 AD) compiled a pharmacopeia containing over 600 plants and plant extracts, including morphine, cocaine, atropine, digitalis, salicylate, ergot, quinine, ephedrine and vinca, all of which are still used in purified forms. His five volume book, *De Materia Medica*, was copied and re-copied until it was first printed in 1478.[7]

Romans employed great efforts to improve the public health system for the good of everyone, regardless of wealth. Part of this policy was driven by the need to ensure that Roman soldiers stayed healthy to maintain the empire.[9]

Romans had an early awareness of bad water and sewage causing ill-health. Consequently their engineering efforts resulted in a sophisticated water supply system, and toilets in houses and streets flushed with running water connected to a sewage system. New cities and military installations were built according to the health of the environment:

> When building a house or farm especial care should be taken to place it at the foot of a wooded hill where it is exposed to health-giving winds. Care should be taken where there are swamps in the neighbourhood, because certain tiny creatures which cannot be seen by the eyes breed there. These float through the air and enter the body by the mouth and nose and cause serious disease.
>
> *Marcus Varro*[9]

> There should be no marshes near buildings, for marshes give off poisonous vapours during the hot period of the summer. At this time, they give birth to animals with mischief-making stings which fly at us in thick swarms.
>
> *Columella*[9]

TOWARDS THE 19TH CENTURY

With the political centre shifting towards Constantinople, medicine was influenced by the Arabic world. Arabic medicine developed new medicines like camphor, saffron, myrrh, musk, iodine, naphtha and senna, and Rhazes (860–952 AD) gave the first description of smallpox.

Cordova in southern Spain became the centre of civilisation around the beginning of the 11th century. Medicine flourished, combining the Hippocratic traditions with the newer knowledge of drugs. The writings of the time influenced the teaching of the medical schools in Renaissance Europe.

Arnold of Villanova (1235–1277) is the father of modern pharmaceuticals. His discovery of the extraction of active ingredients of drugs with alcohol started the refinement of medicines, and the production of tinctures.

SUMMARY POINTS

- The shaman combined three functions: curing the sick, conducting communal sacrifice and escorting the dead to another world.
- Health and illness were constructed from a social perspective.
- Illness was perceived as either a loss of 'soul' or the invasion of destructive external forces.
- One became a shaman/medicine man either by rigorous initiation or formal learning.
- Self-care and folk medicine co-exist with medical care.
- Early medical practice was highly codified and regulated.
- Hippocrates of Cos rejected the notion of supernatural causes of disease, and introduced reasoning and observation into medical practice which formed the basis for the prognosis.
- The Romans introduced public health measures, especially clean water and sanitation, for the good of everyone.

CHAPTER 2

Development of medical knowledge

Where is the life we have lost in living? Where is the wisdom we have lost in knowledge? Where is the knowledge we have lost in information?

TS Eliot[10]

Curiosity is the driving force for the development of knowledge. Since curiosity arises in a particular context, knowledge is neither absolute nor value free. History has shown us how influential these two factors are.

The desire to help pregnant women suffering severe morning sickness led to the discovery of thalidomide, which subsequently was found to have a major risk of causing severe birth defects. The desire to help patients with otherwise difficult to treat conditions has returned attention to the drug. It is now available for the treatment of leprosy, and studies are ongoing to establish its effectiveness in AIDS, autoimmune diseases, macular degeneration and some cancers.[11]

Knowing itself has several dimensions – the information itself, the context it arose from, and the belief system underpinning it. The introduction of thalidomide illustrates this well – the chemical structure and the function of the drug were understood; its development occurred in the context of a common complaint associated with early pregnancy at a time where societal and medical expectation demanded solutions to all complaints.

MILESTONES IN MEDICAL DISCOVERIES

ANATOMY AND PHYSIOLOGY

Man's curiosity to understand his body is an old one. For example trephinations were already routinely conducted between 10 000–5000 BC. The *Ebers papyrus* from 3000 BC describes many diseases including cataracts, haemorrhoids, intestinal parasites, abdominal pain and fractures.

The Greek scientist Alcmaeon of Croton (about 500 BC) dissected cadavers and described the optic nerves. He recognised that the eyes were connected to the brain, and that light had to enter the eye for sight. He also discovered the pharyngotympanic tubes, which later were rediscovered by Eustachius in the 16th century.

Aristotle (384–322 BC) was the first to study comparative anatomy as a way to understand the internal organs of humans. He also is considered to be the father of embryology, having been the first to study the development of the chick embryo.

Herophilus (~300 BC) is regarded as the father of anatomy. At the medical school of Alexandria he vivisected about 600 criminals to study the structure and function of the internal organs.

Galen of Pergamum (131–201 AD) was one of the most influential physicians and anatomists of all time. His work was translated and influenced Persian medicine, and his teachings were still examined by the Royal College of Physicians as late as the end of the 16th century.[12] Galen's outstanding discoveries in anatomy and physiology include such diverse finds as: arteries carry blood, not air; an accurate description of the consequences of spinal cord damage; the diaphragm is not the only muscle involved in breathing; the recurrent laryngeal nerve is responsible for producing voice; and kidneys produce urine.

Leonardo da Vinci (1452–1519) was consumed by his desire to accurately understand the design and function of the human body. He measured every detail he discovered and produced the most accurate anatomical charts of his time.

Andreas Vesalius (1514–1564) corrected many of the misunderstandings of Galenic anatomy, e.g. that the mandible is a single bone, the sternum consists of three parts and that the two ventricles are separated. His book *De Humani Corporis Fabrica* created much controversy as it contradicted the strongly-held beliefs of the time.

In 1628 William Harvey (1578–1657) for the first time accurately described the circulation of blood. He identified that the contraction of the heart pumped blood through the arterial system, and that it subsequently returned back to the heart through the venous system.

POPULATION HEALTH

Major improvements in the health of the community have been achieved by enhancements in nutrition, general hygiene and sanitation in association with improved socioeconomic conditions, and the implementation of population-wide disease prevention programmes.

In 1675, around 8 years after developing a simple microscope that could magnify about 200 times, Anton Leeuwenhoek (1632–1723) discovered bacteria, which laid the foundation for the study of a myriad of infectious diseases.

Edward Jenner (1749–1823), a country doctor, was fascinated by the rural old wives' tale that milkmaids could not get smallpox. Cowpox caused blisters on the hands of milkmaids, and he concluded that the pus in the blisters must protect these women. In 1796, in a daring experiment, he inoculated James Phillips, a small boy, with increasing dosages of pus from the blisters of a milkmaid before deliberately inoculating him with smallpox. James became ill but recovered fully within a few days without developing the disease. His discovery was greeted with great prejudice by the inherently conservative medical establishment in London; however in 1840 the government banned any other than Jenner's treatment for smallpox.

Ignaz Semmelweis (1818–1865) discovered that puerperal fever was caused by cross contamination in hospital wards. In 1847 he introduced vigorous enforcement of strict hand-washing before seeing a pregnant woman, and dramatically reduced the incidence and mortality in his hospital. He also experienced great prejudice from his colleagues, and shortly before his death suffered a nervous breakdown leading to admission to a mental asylum. His observation contradicted the scientific opinion of the time that all diseases were caused by imbalances of basic humours in the body. In addition doctors argued that washing hands before seeing each patient would be too much work, nor were they willing to accept that their own actions could have caused so many deaths.

John Snow (1813–1858), a London surgeon and epidemiologist, made the connection between contaminated drinking water and the outbreak of cholera. In an experiment he removed the handle of the Broad Street pump in Soho, and stopped the epidemic.

These discoveries however, important as they are, are probably not the only reasons for improvement in the health status of the community. As the historical epidemiologist Thomas McKeown (1911–1988) has shown, major improvements in health status over the past 300 years are attributable to improvements in the nutritional status of the population, the improvements in living environments and technologies, improvements in hygiene, drinking water quality and sewage handling, reduction in family size, and the natural change in the virulence and the transmission of disease-causing organisms.[13]

MEDICAL DISCOVERIES

'Modern' medicine, as we understand and practise it today, had its origins in the second half of the 19th century. Technological advances and the systematic development of medical research allowed a detailed study of pathogens and pathology, followed by the development of new therapeutic agents, investigations, and invasive and non-invasive interventions.

Infectious diseases

Louis Pasteur's (1822–1895) suggestion in 1878 that micro-organisms may cause many human and animal diseases – the 'germ theory' – started the discipline of microbiology. He discovered Streptococcus, Staphylococcus and Pneumococcus, and described that rabies was caused by an organism so small (virus) that it could not be seen under the microscope.

Robert Koch (1843–1910) isolated tuberculosis (1882) and cholera (1883), and Edwin Klebs (1834–1913) discovered the diphtheria organism, the three major causes of death of the time.

These findings had immediate impact on the practice of medicine. Though Semmelweis was rejected for his antiseptic techniques, Joseph Lister (1827–1912) successfully introduced them in 1867. Pasteur demonstrated the value of vaccination against anthrax (1879) and rabies (1885), and in 1890 Emil von Behring (1854–1917) and Shibasaburo Kitazato (1852–1931) developed the first effective diphtheria antitoxin.

Pathology

Some pathological changes were already well described as far back as the 15th century, like stomach cancer by the Italian Antonio Benivieni (about 1443–1502), inflammation by John Hunter (1728–1793), or benign and malignant breast disease by Astly Paston Cooper (1768–1841). The major understanding of the relationship between clinical disease and anatomical changes came from the two great pathologists, Carl von Rokitansky (1804–1878) in Vienna, and Rudolf Virchow (1821–1902) in Berlin.

Linking clinical symptoms to post-mortem anatomical changes was first attempted by Battista Morgagni (1682–1771).[14] However, it took more than another 100 years before Rokitansky systematically described and integrated symptoms and pathological changes to diseases, and discussed the consequences of these findings for the diagnostic and therapeutic process. The original publication of incarcerated intestinal hernias should illustrate this:

> Die eigentliche Darmeinschnürung tritt . . . plötzlich mit heftigem Darmschmerz ein, der alsbald den ganzen Unterleib einnimmt, so dass dieser allenthalben höchst empfindlich und schmerzhaft wird. Der Bauch bläht sich allmählich zu einem ungeheuren Volumen auf, wird gespannt, gibt bey Percussion allenthalben einen hellen Darmton . . . Dagegen ist häufiges Erbrechen zugegen . . . Was die Therapie betrifft, so verlässt uns . . . jede Arznei . . . [es] lässt sich – offen gestanden – nicht wohl ein anderes Mittel ersinnen, die Darmeinschnürung zu heben, als das Messer (Rokitansky C (1836) Über innere Darmeinschnürungen Medizinische Jahrbücher des k.k. österreichischen Staates NF19, S 632–676).[15]

> [The obstruction occurs suddenly, starting with severe bowel pain and soon affecting the whole abdomen which becomes extremely sensitive and painful. The abdomen distends slowly to become huge and tense, and hyper-resonant to percussion. Frequent vomiting is present . . . In terms of therapy every known medicine fails us – and quite frankly – I cannot think of any other way to treat the incarceration but to use the knife.]

The suggestion to operate on an incarcerated bowel created much discussion since the accepted standard treatment at the time was the frequent application of enemas.

Virchow demonstrated the cellular changes of disease. He observed that every cell is derived from a cell (*Omnis cellula e cellula*) which was the basis for the 'cell theory of disease' and the foundation of cellular pathology. His thinking still influences today's research paradigm.

Diagnostic imaging

During 1895 Wilhelm Roentgen (1845–1923) discovered the X-ray beam, and the first medical X-ray taken in February 1896 allowed the non-invasive diagnosis of disease in the living. This started the revolution of new diagnostic possibilities.

In 1956 Prof Ian Donald (1910–1987) performed the first obstetric ultrasound examination in Glasgow, and since the development of computer tomography (CT scan) by Godfrey Hounsfield (1919–2004) in 1972, diagnostic accuracy has been greatly enhanced. In 1975 Richard Ernst (born 1933) proposed magnetic resonance imaging (MRI), but it took till 1986 for the technology to become fast enough to be introduced into routine clinical practice. Further enhancements have led to the development of functional MRI which allows the study of biochemical processes within tissues and organs.

Pharmacotherapy

Pharmaceutical drugs greatly advanced the management of many diseases, none more so than the discovery of the anaesthetic agents ether by Crawford Long (1815–1878) in 1842, and nitrous oxide by Horace Wells (1815–1848) in 1844.

Hippocrates used a powder from the bark and leaves of the willow tree to relieve pain and fever. In 1829 scientists discovered the active compound, salicin. Raffaele Piria (1814–1865) purified salicin to salicylic acid. It was highly effective but very tough on the stomach. The buffering of salicylic acid to acetylsalicylic acid by Charles Gerhard overcame the problem. Gerhard didn't market his discovery, and it was Felix Hoffmann (1867–1946), a chemist working for Bayer in Germany, who rediscovered the compound, and by 1899 had convinced the company to commercially release it under the name of aspirin.

One of the great pharmaceutical breakthroughs was the extraction of insulin by Frederick Banting (1891–1941) in 1921, a discovery that improved and saved the lives of many.

Protonsil, the first sulfa drug discovered by Gerhard Domagk (1895–1964) in 1935, was also the first antibiotic used in clinical practice for the treatment of streptococcal infection. Though Alexander Fleming (1881–1955) had discovered penicillin seven years earlier, it took until 1941 before Howard Florey (1898–1968) and Ernst Chain (1906–1979) introduced it into clinical practice, achieving the successful treatment of many infectious diseases. 1944 saw the discovery of streptomycin, the first effective treatment against tuberculosis by Selman Waksman (1888–1973).

Other important drugs include diuretics, which were already known to Paracelsus (mercurous chloride), and digitalis which is known for more than 200 years. Important specific and potent drugs introduced in the last 50 years include beta-blockers and angiotensin-converting enzyme (ACE)-inhibitors, H_2-blockers – cimetidine was introduced in 1979 – and proton pump inhibitors (PPIs) for gastric ulcers, and immuno-suppressives for the treatment of a range of autoimmune diseases and in transplantation medicine.

Other important discoveries and breakthroughs

1952 saw the development of the cardiac pacemaker by Paul Zoll (1911–1999); in 1953 James Watson (born 1928) and Francis Crick (1916–2004) discovered the double helix structure of DNA, which paved the way for medical genetics and the human genome project; in the 1950s artificial joint replacement was pioneered by Frederick Thompson,

Austin Moore and John Charnley (1911–1982); fibre-optic sigmoidoscopy was developed by Bergein Overholt (born 1938) in 1963; the first successful heart transplantation was performed by Christiaan Barnard (1922–2001) in 1967; and in 1977 Andreas Gruentzig (1939–1985) performed the first coronary angioplasty.

THE BEGINNINGS OF EPIDEMIOLOGY

There is no exact birth date of epidemiology as a science, and a web search shows that the definition of epidemiology contains some variability: 'The study of disease in human populations' (web.mit.edu/environment/ehs/topic/ HazCommTerms.html); 'The branch of medical science dealing with the transmission and control of disease' (wordnet. princeton.edu/perl/webwn); 'The study of disease in populations. These studies relate the incidence and prevalence of disease to genetic and environmental factors' (cll.ucsd. edu/glossarye.htm).

Looking backwards one has to acknowledge the epidemiological understanding of Jenner, Semmelweis and Snow, well before Pasteur and Koch could demonstrate the causative agents of the various disease outbreaks.

Bacteriology and epidemiology historically are closely linked, and the focus of understanding disease outbreaks was more bacteriologically focused in Germany, compared to the pursuit of environmental factors in the UK and the US.[16]

The germ theory of disease proved all pervasive – starting from Snow who postulated it *a priori*, to Koch who provided the evidence. Nevertheless there were doubters about the simple cause and effect relationship between organisms and disease, the most famous being Max von Pettenkofer (1818–1901), a German public health physician, who raised the question of whether it was sufficient to have the organism present or did one also need to have co-factors in the host and the environment? von Pettenkofer was famous for his – later largely disproved – 'Boden theory' postulating a multifactorial mechanism of environmental factors in the soil causing disease. To prove his *multifactorial* theory and to disprove the simple *cause-and-effect* principle postulated by the germ theory, he and some famous co-investigators of his time drank cholera broth without getting sick.[17]

von Pettenkofer was proved wrong despite his successful experiment; however, his main notion – the multifactorial nature of disease and illness – after all turned out to be correct.[18] Differentiating between causality and correlation amongst potential risk variables remains a difficult, and at times contentious, issue.

IMPORTANT EPIDEMIOLOGICAL STUDIES OF THE 20TH CENTURY

In 1948 the Medical Research Council (MRC) in the UK alerted researchers to the huge increase in lung cancer and asked if this increase is real, and if so, what the underlying cause may be. Smoking was regarded as a normal and harmless habit, and 80% of men smoked. It was believed that the increase in air pollution from coal fires, cars and industry was responsible. Richard Doll (1912–2005) and Bradford Hill (1897–1991) conducted a brief questionnaire survey amongst 650 patients admitted to a London hospital with suspected lung, liver and bowel cancer, as well as hospital patients admitted with other diagnoses. Those finally diagnosed with lung cancer overwhelmingly were smokers, those cleared non-smokers.[19]

The findings were so compelling but so unexpected that Doll and Hill sought advice on their findings from the head of the MRC, Harold Himsworth. He considered that the findings may be peculiar to London and suggested the study was repeated in other towns; the same results were revealed. Richard Doll valued this advice and stated:

> It was a principle that I have adhered to ever since: namely, that if you find something that is unexpected and is going to be of social significance you have a responsibility to be sure that you're right before you publicise your results to the rest of the world. This does at least require repeating some of your observations.[20]

The Framingham Heart Study is the longest longitudinal community study in the world. It was set up in 1948 to investigate the leading cause of death and serious illness in the US (and the Western world) – cardiovascular disease. At the time little was known about the causes of heart disease. The aim of the study was to seek out the common factors leading to the disease in as-yet asymptomatic people. The key findings of the study are presented in Box 2.1.

The study started with 5209 men and women between the ages of 30 and 62 years, from the town of Framingham, Massachusetts, and in 1971 was extended to involve a second generation, the offspring cohort consisting of 5124 adult children and their spouses from the original study group. The study is now recruiting a further 3500 grandchildren of the original cohort.[21]

BOX 2.1   The highlights of the Framingham Heart Study[21]

1956	Findings on the progression of rheumatic heart disease
1959	Factors found that increase the likelihood of heart disease
1960	Cigarette smoking found to increase the risk of heart disease
1961	Cholesterol level, blood pressure, and electrocardiogram abnormalities found to increase the risk of heart disease
1967	Physical activity found to reduce the risk of heart disease and obesity to increase the risk of heart disease
1970	High blood pressure found to increase the risk of stroke
1974	Overview of diabetes and its complications
1976	Menopause found to increase the risk of heart disease
1977	Effects of triglycerides and low-density lipoprotein (LDL) and high-density lipoprotein (HDL) cholesterol described
1978	Psychosocial factors found to affect heart disease
	Atrial fibrillation (condition in which the heart beats irregularly) found to increase the risk of stroke
1981	Filter cigarettes found to give no protection against coronary heart disease
	Major report issued on the relationship of diet and heart disease

1983   Reports on mitral valve prolapse (which causes a backward leak of blood between heart chambers)

1988   High levels of HDL cholesterol found to reduce risk of death

Type 'A' behaviour associated with heart disease

Isolated systolic hypertension found to increase risk of heart disease

Cigarette smoking found to increase risk of stroke

1990   Homocysteine (an amino acid) found as a possible risk factor for heart disease

1991   Heart disease risk prediction models produced

1993   Mild isolated systolic hypertension shown to increase the risk of heart disease

Major report predicts survival after diagnosis of heart failure

1994   Enlarged left ventricle (one of two lower chambers of the heart) shown to increase the risk of stroke

Lipoprotein (a) found as a possible risk factor for heart disease

Risk factors for atrial fibrillation described

Apolipoprotein E found as possible risk factor for heart disease

1995   First Framingham report on diastolic heart failure

1996   Progression from hypertension to heart failure described

1997   Report on the cumulative effects of smoking and high cholesterol on the risk for atherosclerosis

Investigation of the impact of an enlarged left ventricle and risk for heart failure in asymptomatic individuals

FROM A SLOW START

Figures 2.1 and 2.2 compress the history of medicine on a logarithmic scale. The philosophical assumptions, the knowledge base and the practice of medicine had changed little till the end of the Middle Ages. The 17th century saw the start of the scientific revolution, initially enhancing anatomical understanding, and during the 19th century the discovery of the causes of disease; the 20th century accelerated both, our knowledge and our management based on the application of ever more sophisticated technology.

The changes in knowledge and the changes in the practice of medicine caused major crises in the self-understanding of the medical profession, ultimately resulting in the fragmentation along particular aspects of the human body with the exception of the general practitioner/family physician who always embraced the whole person.

DEVELOPMENT OF MEDICAL KNOWLEDGE

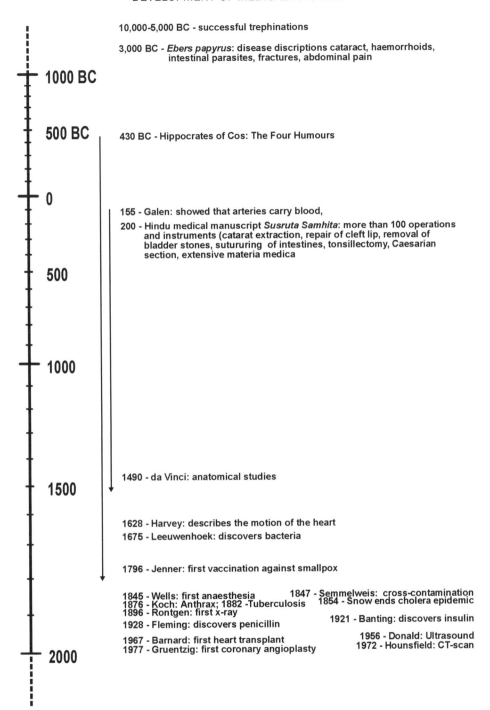

Figure 2.1 The acceleration of medical discoveries.

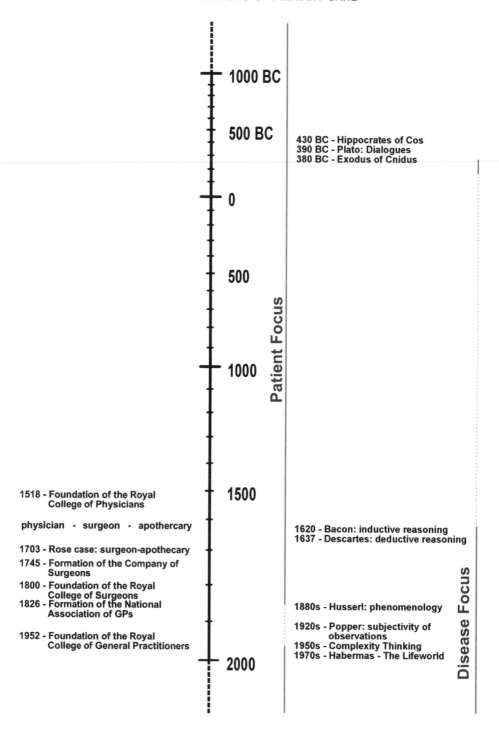

Figure 2.2 The progression of philosophical understandings and professional evolution.

SUMMARY POINTS

- Knowledge is neither absolute nor value free.
- Anatomical studies informed the understanding of medicine until the 17th century.
- Astute observation was the basis for understanding endemic diseases like smallpox and puerperal fever.
- Observations that contradicted current beliefs or practices were treated with great prejudice.
- Improvements in nutrition, hygiene, drinking water and disposal of sewage were more important in improving the health status of the community than improvements in medical knowledge and practice.
- Pasteur's germ theory of disease dominated medical thinking and laid the foundation for bacteriology.
- Rokitansky correlated symptoms and pathology to inform management.
- Virchow's cellular theory of disease advanced the understanding of all disease, and is still influencing today's research paradigm.
- 20th century technological development accelerated the understanding, detection and treatment of many diseases.
- Epidemiology studies the origins of diseases in the population, and has identified that many diseases have multifactorial causes.

CHAPTER 3

The history of medical education

I taught medicine at the bedside.

Sir William Osler [22]

The history of medical education in ancient times is not that clear, but in general terms it was largely apprenticeship based in Greece, Byzantium and Egypt. In early Roman times medicine was not organised in any particular way, and the standing of the physician in society was low. There were no formal requirements for the entrance to the profession; anyone could call himself a doctor. If his methods were successful, he attracted more patients; if not, he found himself another profession.

Until recently, Diaulus was a doctor; now he is an undertaker. He is still doing as an undertaker, what he used to do as a doctor.

Martial, Epigrams 1.47 [23]

Galen's influence on medical thinking and medical education prevailed for almost 1500 years. He also greatly influenced medical education by insisting that besides developing medical skills, the training of a doctor must include the study of philosophy, immortalising this conviction in his treatise *That the best Doctor is also a Philosopher*. This tradition lasted well into the Renaissance.

The Salerno School flourished during the 9th to 13th centuries, and was the first one that had a final examination. Graduates called themselves 'doctor' – the learned one – rather than the traditional 'medicus'.[7]

MEDICAL EDUCATION IN THE RENAISSANCE

Three famous Italian medical educators of the Renaissance all stressed that the physician must have a broad education emphasising social and environmental awareness and practical competence, knowledge and intellectual ability, and broad culture.

Girolamo Cardano (1501–1576) insisted that

> ... medicine requires and encompasses mastery of almost all forms of technical knowledge and practical wisdom: astrology, meteorology (for the effects of climate), architecture and cookery (for the effects of housing and diet), natural history, natural magic, medicinal botany and pharmacology, anatomy, prophecy (in the form of prognostication), and even theology, for the physician's contemplation of life and death, soul and body, brings him close to the divine.[24]

Paduan professor Gian Battista Da Monte (1498–1551) saw the

> ... prerequisites for success in medicine as he knew it were verbal and ratiocinative: an aptitude for discussion and speculation, and a knowledge of logic and philosophy.[24]

Girolamo Mercuriale (1530–1606) put it more simply:

> 'read "poets and historians" along with [your] medical textbooks'.[24]

A university degree in medicine consisted of theoretical study, supplemented with practical instruction, and was a recognised qualification and a prerequisite to entering the College of Physicians. It also provided the authority to supervise other practitioners.

MEDICAL EDUCATION IN EUROPE

At the beginning of the 18th century, the Vienna medical school was hardly active, with the appointed professors rarely giving lectures or writing texts for their students. In addition the university received little money to maintain its infrastructure. In 1745 Empress Maria Theresia promoted Gerard van Swieten (1700–1772) to reform the university and in particular the medical school. Under his leadership the new university was built, and the salary for professors was increased generously to allow them to concentrate solely on their teaching and academic duties.

Van Swieten was educated in the famous school at Leyden. He reduced lecture-based instruction substantially and introduced the Dutch bedside teaching model to Vienna. His colleague Anton de Haën (1704–1776) instructed his students at the bedside as well as at post-mortem examinations, demonstrating the correlations of clinical signs and the effects of treatments, the beginning of comparative pathology.

In 1775 van Swieten's pupil, Anton Störck (1731–1803), proposed a major reform plan for the medical school which divided the course into preliminary studies of botany, chemistry and physiology, then pathology and materia medica (pharmacology), followed by clinical studies in the hospital. The plan received royal endorsement and formed the basic organisation of European medical schools until today.

MEDICAL EDUCATION IN AMERICA AND THE FLEXNER REPORT

Modern medical education in the Western world is based on the Flexnerian model. Abraham Flexner, in his 1910 report on medical education in the US and Canada (*see* Box 3.1),[25] describes the historical developments, starting with the apprenticeship model of the 17th and 18th century as follows:

> The likely youth of that period, destined to a medical career, was at an early age indentured to some reputable practitioner, to whom his service was successively menial, pharmaceutical, and professional: he ran his master's errands, washed the bottles, mixed the drugs, spread the plasters, and finally, as the stipulated term drew towards its close, actually took part in the daily practice of his preceptor – bleeding his patients, pulling their teeth, and obeying a hurried summons in the night. The quality of the training varied within large limits with the capacity and conscientiousness of the master.[25] (p. 3)

In the 1750s the American medical school was conceived as an educational enterprise between the university and the teaching hospital, based on the realisation that the students

> ... must Join Examples with Study, before he can be sufficiently qualified to prescribe for the sick, for Language and Books alone can never give him Adequate Ideas of Diseases and the best methods of Treating them, ... There the Clinical professor comes in to the Aid of Speculation and demonstrates the Truth of Theory by Facts, he meets his pupils at stated times in the Hospital, and when a case presents adapted to his purpose, he asks all those Questions which lead to a certain knowledge of the Disease and parts Affected; and if the Disease baffles the power of Art and the Patient falls a Sacrifice to it, he then brings his Knowledge to the Test, and fixes Honour or discredit on his Reputation by exposing all the Morbid parts to View, and Demonstrates by what means it produced Death, and if perchance he finds something unexpected, which Betrays an Error in Judgement, he like a great and good man immediately acknowledges the mistake, and, for the benefit of survivors, points out other methods by which it might have been more happily treated.[25] (p. 4)

However the courses varied widely in structure, content and quality – many left a medical programme frankly unqualified. Flexner adhered to the firmly held view that medicine is a scientific enterprise, and that learning medicine requires prior knowledge of biology, chemistry and physics, without which, he concluded, the education of the medical student would be suboptimal.

However Flexner also appreciated the humanistic side of medicine, and the changing role of the doctor in society:

> ... he needs a different apperceptive and appreciative apparatus to deal with other, more subtle elements ... one must rely for the requisite insight and sympathy on a varied and

enlarging cultural experience. Such enlargement of the physician's horizon is otherwise important, for scientific progress has greatly modified his ethical responsibility . . . But the physician's function is fast becoming social and preventive, rather than individual and curative . . . Upon him society relies to ascertain, and through measures essentially educational to enforce, the conditions that prevent disease and make positively for physical and moral wellbeing. It goes without saying that this type of doctor is first of all an educated man.[25] (p. 26)

BOX 3.1 Contents page: *The Flexner Report* – Part I

Chapter I	Historical and General
Chapter II	The Proper Basis of Medical Education
Chapter III	The Actual Basis of Medical Education
Chapter IV	The Course of Study: The Laboratory Branches
Chapter V	The Course of Study: The Laboratory Branches – cont
Chapter VI	The Course of Study: The Hospital and the Medical School
Chapter VII	The Course of Study: The Hospital and the Medical School – cont
Chapter VIII	The Financial Aspects of Medical Education
Chapter IX	Reconstruction
Chapter X	The Medical Sects
Chapter XI	The State Boards
Chapter XII	The Postgraduate School
Chapter XIII	The Medical Education for Women
Chapter XIV	The Medical Education of the Negro

Flexner proposed a universal postgraduate programme for all medical schools consisting of a two-year science-based component – anatomy, physiology, pharmacology and pathology, followed by a two-year clinical programme – medicine, surgery and obstetrics. Not only was Flexner concerned with the structure and the content of the programme, he also had firm views on the means of instruction.

On the pedagogic side, modern medicine, like all scientific teaching, is characterized by activity. The student no longer merely watches, listens, memorizes; he does. His own activities in the laboratory and in the clinic are the main factors in his instruction and discipline. An education in medicine nowadays involves both learning and learning how; the student cannot effectively know, unless he knows how.[25] (p. 53)

The student's clinical work is classified under four heads: (1) medicine, in which pediatrics and infectious disease may be included, (2) surgery, (3) obstetrics, (4) the specialities, such as diseases of the eye, ear, skin, etc. A teaching hospital consists essentially of a series or wards, accommodating patients belonging to these several departments, each ward systematically organized . . .[25] (p. 94)

CONSEQUENCES OF THE FLEXNER REFORMS

Flexner's reforms were certainly needed at a time of fragmented and substandard medical education.[26] His personal preference for allopathic treatment shaped his recommendations for the medical curriculum,[27] and consequently shaped the direction of the research agenda almost exclusively towards the natural sciences, to the detriment of all other forms of enquiry into the human conditions of disease and illness. On the positive side, Flexner had a holistic view about the role of medicine, he clearly saw – and articulated – the need for a change in the role of the doctor, as well as the need to unify the foundations of medicine within a scientific framework. Unfortunately, medical schools focused most of their energy on implementing the science-based components into their medical programmes, and based them within the hospital setting, thus paving the way for medicine to become a technology [28,29] and

> . . . to separate the disease from the man and the man from his environment.[28]

Not surprisingly these changes very soon showed their 'unintended consequences', as Crookshank remarked in the *Lancet* in 1926:

> It is in sympathy with this attitude towards inquiry into the mental processes by which we obtain our 'facts' that all traces of metaphysics, logic, and philosophy has [sic] disappeared from medical education since in becoming more medical, it became less educative[30]

and Flexner himself, a keen observer of the progress in medical education, commented with some regret, particularly about the fragmentation of care and the deterioration of the doctor–patient relationship:

> . . . the very intensity with which scientific medicine is cultivated threatens to cost us at times the mellow judgement and broad culture of the older generation at its best. Osler, Janeway, and Halsted have not been replaced.[31]

The deficiencies of hospital-based training, both before and after Flexner's reforms have been most evident in general practice/family medicine. Sir James Mackenzie wrote about his experience after starting in general practice in 1879:

> After a year in hospital as house physician, I entered general practice in an industrial town of about 100 000 inhabitants. I started my work fairly confident that my teaching, and hospital experience, had amply furnished me with competent knowledge for the pursuit of my profession . . . I was not long engaged in my new sphere when I realized that I was unable to recognize the ailments in the great majority of my patients. (cited in reference 28)

The impact of the scientific and technological emphasis of 20th century medical education are succinctly summarised by McWhinney:

Although the understanding of patients and their illnesses requires a blend of objective and subjective knowledge, medical education has become concerned overwhelmingly with objective knowledge. The *episteme* of technology has become the *episteme* of medicine.[29]

NEW APPROACHES TO MEDICAL EDUCATION

[Medicine is] an old art [that] . . . must be absorbed in the new sciences.

Sir William Osler[26]

The Flexner-based medical curriculum had an unchallenged run until the early 1980s. Some of the criticisms about the performance of medical schools are exemplified in comments by McWhinney in 1975:

> In his essay on the educational ideas of Coleridge, William Walsh describes modern education as being 'under the dominance of the foreground, the sustained and peremptory dominance of subject-matter'. Subject matter, the readily accessible, examinable information 'has distended to monstrous proportions, monstrous in its immensity, shapelessness and horrid incoherence'. Yet how little of this foreground remains and influences the remainder of one's life? A good education transcends subject matter . . . 'A good education persists not as a collection of information, an arrangement of intellectual bric-a-brac, but a certain unity of self . . . and a certain method of thinking and feeling' . . . Of critical importance, certainly, is the setting of education. If students are to have certain values and certain ways of thinking and feeling, they must be educated in a setting in which these qualities are all-pervasive.[28]

Louden in 1983:

> In the modern university, abstraction and disengaged reason reign supreme. Knowledge has been separated from experience, thinking from feeling. The educational challenge we face is correcting, in Margaret Donaldson's words, 'the imbalance between intellectual and emotional development'. In medicine, the standard diagnostic method is an outstanding example of the imbalance. The physician is required to categorize the illness, but not to attend to the patient's feelings or understand his experience.[32]

and McCormick in 1993:

> Medical school education is authoritarian, and examinations require regurgitation of what are essentially ex cathedra statements . . . the failure of medical education to cultivate science as a way of thought and to encourage and fertilize the growth of 'scepticaemia' has serious consequences for the well-being of our patients.[5]

Three emerging themes characterise the failings of the educational system – an unsuitable (hospital) learning environment, the predominant focus on subject matter fails to teach the connexial dimension with our patients, the basis for the healing relationship, and the critical attitude towards the doctrines of the day.

Medical education is a socialising process that occurs in the clinical context. Students require early positive experiences, especially within the primary and community care environment, and within an apprenticeship situation to become confident in dealing with patients and other healthcare providers.[26]

COMMUNITY-BASED LEARNING

The ideas of problem-based learning as a strategy, and learning in the community as the better learning environment, emerged simultaneously in the early 1980s. Both were seen as providing lifelong learning strategies.

> The core curriculum for all doctors should be primary care: this should be taught where it is actually carried out, within communities; and the primary generalists produced in this way require not a year or two of rehabilitation in specialized vocational training, but a lifetime of in-service postgraduate study.[33]

The first successful attempts at community-based medical education occurred at the University of New Mexico School of Medicine,[34,35] the University of Gezira, Egypt,[36] and the Upper Peninsula Medical Education Program at Michigan State University.[37] These programmes have been adapted in many countries, and more recently some attempts have been made to expand this approach to the entire clinical curriculum, though mostly in rural settings.[38,39]

PATIENT-CENTRED LEARNING

Community-based medical education has been a major step forward both by providing a better learning environment and as a response to changing community needs. However in large parts it has not put the patient at the centre of the learning effort. Patient-centred learning incorporates this aspect, a concern already expressed by McWhinney in 1975:

> What kind of people, then, do educators want their students to become? They should have a deep commitment to people and obtain their greatest professional fulfilment from their relations with people – to believe, in Lewis Mumford's phrase, in the primacy of the person, to use technology with skill, but to make it always subservient to the interests of the person. Educators want physicians who can think analytically when analysis is required but whose usual mode of thought is multi-dimensional and holistic. They want them to be concerned with aetiology in its broadest sense to be ever mindful of the need to teach their patients how to attain and maintain health. They want people who are not afraid of recognizing and talking about feelings: people who know themselves and can throughout their career recognize their defects, learn from experience and continue to grow as people and as physicians.[28]

Patient-centred medicine firstly sees the patient as a person,[29] aims to understand the

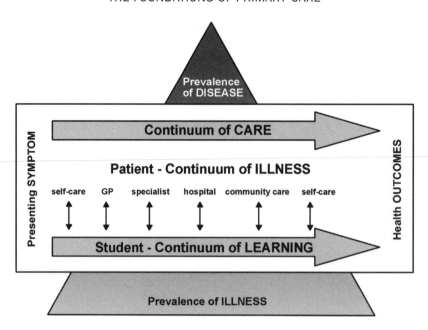

Figure 3.1   The longitudinal patient-centred model of clinical education.

human impact of the illness experience of every patient in its unique ways,[40] and stands in contrast to the traditional largely disease-focused 20th century approach.

One such model of teaching has been developed and successfully implemented in rural Australia.[41] The concept of this particular programme assumed that patients present with troublesome symptoms – rather than a diagnosis – and that holistic learning requires students to have continuity with *their* patients, hence they accompany them on their journey through the healthcare system. Students directly experience the complexities of suddenly being a patient, having to navigate the healthcare system, and most profoundly having to *make sense* of and adapt to being ill. The emphasis here is on *illness*, since illness can exist in the absence of disease, and yet illness requires medical care. Having shared their patients' journey through the healthcare system provides them with transformational, i.e. deep, learning experiences and growth (*see* Figure 3.1).[42] Having had the opportunity to reflect they gain knowledge about *the how* in addition to *the why* an illness affects a patient in a particular way.

ONGOING CHALLENGES

On a broad scale, medical education has to resolve two issues which are partly educationally and partly politically driven.

The first is the distinction between *educating* and *training* doctors. The former will lead to integrated human and technical *capabilities* based on an understanding of the patient; the latter will lead to focused and technical *competence* based on understanding 'predefined' diseases. Some medical courses have decided to aim for a capability approach – Box 3.2 provides an example from the University of New South Wales, Australia.[43]

BOX 3.2 Student capabilities: University of New South Wales[43]

Applied knowledge and skills

1 Using basic and clinical sciences in medical practice
   - explains mechanisms that maintain a state of health
   - describes pathophysiology of diseases and explains at whole person, organ, cellular and molecular levels
   - anticipates complications and their basis
   - plans and justifies appropriate investigations
   - explains how management plans alter the illness or disease process

2 Understanding the social determinants of health and disease
   - identifies social and cultural factors that contribute to health or illness
   - collaborates with other healthcare professionals in health promotion and disease prevention
   - is able to refer patients to community-based healthcare services and collaborates appropriately

3 Patient assessment and management
   - identifies social, cultural and psychological factors that impact on a patient's health
   - handles unexpected findings and prolonged uncertainty appropriately
   - conducts a proficient examination related to the patient and their presentation
   - demonstrates effective clinical reasoning and diagnostic skills in response to clinical problems
   - recognises typical and atypical features of a presentation
   - procedural skills

Interactional abilities

4 Effective communication
   - conducts proficient in-depth consultation
   - communicates effectively across a clinical team

5 Working as a member of a team
   - recognises the significant features of a team, including roles, responsibilities, personalities and power relations
   - analyses events in a team from others' viewpoints, including identifying their goals and recognising their feelings
   - analyses and solves problems collaboratively, behaves pro-actively, taking action and responsibility when necessary

Personal attributes

6 Self-directed learning and critical evaluation skills
   - identifies own learning needs and undertakes appropriate formal and informal educational activities routinely
   - identifies future postgraduate learning needs, environments and challenges; develops strategies and skills to facilitate transition to subsequent training

BOX 3.2 *cont.*

7 Understanding and acting in an ethical and socially responsible manner
- articulates personal and professional values
- understands and can discuss a number of different ethical perspectives and apply these to clinical situations
- recognises the complexity of ethical issues throughout all stages of life and responds appropriately and with consideration for the needs of patients and their families
- analyses the extent that systems and institutional procedures support equitable and compassionate health care

8 Development as a reflective practitioner
- recognises and takes into account the influence of contextual, social, political and cultural factors, and the viewpoints of others, when discussing issues, or when formulating and justifying clinical plans and actions
- develops plans for action and for coping in potentially difficult and/or stressful situations
- responds flexibly to changing and uncertain situations
- recognises the limits of his/her own and others' knowledge and skill, and seeks appropriate and timely assistance
- acknowledges his or her limitations and mistakes, and reflects on them so as to develop both personally and professionally

The other is linked to the first and relates to the general structure and the length of medical courses. The worldwide trend to postgraduate courses for medicine on the one hand attracts more mature students and students from diverse backgrounds, on the other, despite compressing the main clinical experience into often only 2 or 3 years, it still lengthens the overall length of study and thus impacts negatively on the supply of doctors to the community at a time of a rapidly rising doctor shortage. McWhinney for example cautions:

> Medicine being a practical craft skill demands the re-introduction of the apprenticeship model of learning, and teachers need to be clinical craftsman rather than simply masters of science or teaching. Since the acquisition of craft skills require time, one carefully has to consider the consequences of shortening undergraduate and postgraduate training programmes, and in particular the early entry into specialisation.[29]

The compression of the medical course into a shorter timeframe threatens the apprenticeship model of learning; after all, working with the master over time enables the novice to learn and gain confidence in the craft. Medical education has to balance the biomedical needs in the context of a wider framework; today that wider framework includes clinical environments in the community that offer practical clinical experiences relevant to the needs of doctors in the 21st century. Dornan explored these requirements which are summarised the Table 3.1.[26]

TABLE 3.1 Enhancing apprenticeship-based learning[26]

PREREQUISITES FOR TRADITIONAL APPRENTICESHIP	CONSTRAINTS IN CURRENT HEALTHCARE SYSTEM	POSSIBLE SOLUTIONS
Clinician-teachers		
Breadth	Narrowness	Avoid overspecialisation in secondary care, and offer apprenticeships in primary as well as secondary care
Integrated practice	Specialisation	
Continuity of supervision	Discontinuity	Mentorship
Time	Lack of time	Make sessional commitments to teaching explicit
Teaching accorded high priority	Teaching below service delivery, administration and research in priority	Develop promotion tracks for education
Themselves trained by apprenticeship	Lack of an apprenticeship tradition	Faculty development
Learning environment		
Uniprofessional and collegial	Multiprofessional	Capitalise on multiprofessional teams for apprenticeship learning
Personal	Impersonal	Personalise attachments as far as possible, and make them long enough for learners and teachers to get to know one another
Person focused	Technology focused	
Space for students	No space	Give students a base close to where care is delivered
Students living on-site	Students and staff live off-site	Organise residential apprenticeship attachments
Patients		
On hospital wards	More care in outpatient department and community	Deliver it in ambulatory as well as inpatient settings
A rich case mix	Less gross organic disease, more psychosocial illness	Teach 'patient-centred care' that acknowledges the experience of illness as well as the disease process
Long stays	Short stays, if admitted at all	Follow episodes of illness across the primary/secondary care interface
Students		
Manageable numbers	Huge expansion in numbers	Disperse learning and ensure individual mentorship

SUMMARY POINTS

- Doctor means 'the learned one'.
- Medical education always emphasised an understanding of all knowledge domains.
- Bedside teaching started in the medical school of Padua in the 16th century.
- The Vienna Medical School, in the late 18th century, introduced the division of medical education into a pre-clinical and clinical component.
- 1910, Abraham Flexner laid the foundations of the structure of medical schools and medical education around the world, based on his understanding of medicine as a scientific endeavour.
- Flexner also highlighted the humanistic and social qualities of the doctor; however these aspects got lost in the implementation of his reforms.
- Flexner's ideology propelled the understanding of diseases and their management, but also virtually squashed any other enquiry into the human experience of disease and illness.
- 20 years after his report Flexner expressed his concerns about the fragmentation of care and the deterioration of the doctor–patient relationship.
- The problematic areas of medical in the 21st century remain the predominance of the teaching hospital, the predominant teaching focus on subject matter in preference to the development of the 'self' of the student, and the lack of broad critical appraisal of the belief systems of the day.
- Medical education must focus on integrating the human and technical capabilities based on an understanding of the patient, a concept distinctively different from the prevailing focus on training the technical competencies required to deal with predefined diseases.

CHAPTER 4

The origins of general practice/family medicine

A pessimist sees the difficulty in every opportunity; an optimist sees the opportunity in every difficulty.

Winston Churchill

THE STRUGGLE FOR RECOGNITION

The origins of general practice/family medicine as a distinct discipline and the general practitioner/family physician as a distinct medical person are somewhat nebulous. The term *practitioner* was not used prior to 1800. At that time three different professions practised medicine – the university-educated physician who dealt with internal disorders; the surgeon, a craftsman, who dealt with external disorders and conditions requiring manual interventions; and the tradesman apothecary who dispensed the physician's prescriptions.

General practice/family medicine as a discipline emerged in the UK. In 1703–1704 the House of Lords (Upper House of Parliament in the UK) in its Rose case decision granted apothecaries the right to 'practise physic', i.e. to visit, to advise and to prescribe, but only to charge for the medicines prescribed. Over time a group of practitioners started to deliberately practise medicine, surgery, midwifery and pharmacy – the birth of the general practitioner, as they were known by 1840.

The beginnings of the general practitioner era in the UK were tumultuous, and in a way not that dissimilar from the tensions encountered today. In 1812 Anthony Todd Thompson (1778–1849) seized the moment to protest against the increasing tax on apothecaries and surgeon-apothecaries – a very high tax applied to glass and was used to finance the war, and founded the first general practitioners' association, the Association of Apothecaries and Surgeon-Apothecaries. The association proposed a bill to regulate the medical profession – future general practitioners would attend a newly founded medical school, be examined and licensed to practise medicine, surgery and midwifery by a 'fourth body', they hoped would be started by members of the association, and required to hold the diploma of membership of the Royal College of Surgeons.

The plan was successfully rejected by the reactionary and self-centred Colleges of Physicians and Surgeons. In 1815 a greatly weakened bill was passed that required general practitioners to undergo a five-year apprenticeship before presenting for licensing by the Society of Apothecaries – the group who was given the task despite not asking for it – followed by a six-month period of practice at a recognised hospital or dispensary. The majority of general practitioners also obtained the Diploma of the Royal College of Surgeons. This outcome was highly unsatisfactory, and despite many efforts the Association of Apothecaries and Surgeon-Apothecaries failed to alter the act and dissolved itself in 1827.

Nevertheless the new arrangements were effective in training and licensing new general practitioners, most of them coming from the rising middle class, and the number of practitioners grew very fast, in fact so fast that the profession was overcrowded, and many were unable to make a living out of it – in England there was one general practitioner per 1000 people compared with one per 2200 in 1970.

The failures of these early years meant that general practitioners were out there on their own, without any body, and without any opportunities to meet and consult with each other. In 1844 Robert Rainey Pennington (1764–1849) founded the National Association of General Practitioners with the aim of establishing the Royal College of General Practitioners in Medicine, Surgery and Midwifery. Within months it had 4000 members, representing about 30% of all general practitioners in England and Wales.

The National Association presented a simple plan for the registration of all doctors, a preliminary examination by physicians and surgeons for all those wishing to enter the medical profession followed by a period of study in medicine, surgery or general practice. Final registration would follow a second examination by the appropriate college; general practitioners would have been trained and examined by their own peers.

Again the Colleges of Physicians and Surgeons had many objections to the plan. After prolonged negotiations it was finally agreed that the order of examinations would be reversed for general practitioners; the final examination would be conducted by physicians and surgeons. In 1848 at a joint conference between the National Institute of Medicine, Surgery and Midwifery (the old National Association), the Colleges of Physicians and Surgeons and the Society of Apothecaries agreement for the foundation of a College of General Practitioners was reached. However at the eleventh hour the College of Surgeons backed away from the agreement.[44]

THE FORMATION OF THE COLLEGES OF GENERAL PRACTICE

General practice lingered on for the next 100 years, having no formal structure and organisation. In fact many general practitioners in the UK felt very disenfranchised, and morale was very low. Joseph Collings, a visiting Australian general practitioner invited by the Nuffield Provincial Hospital Trust in 1948, described his impressions in the *Lancet*:

> There are no real standards for general practice. What the doctor does, and how he does it, depends almost wholly on his own conscience.
>
> The conduct of general practice and of the individual practitioner is inextricably interwoven with commercial and emotional considerations, which too often negate the code of medical ethics by which the public are supposedly safeguarded and from which the high reputation of medicine stems.
>
> An attempt should be made to define the future province and function of general practice within the frame work of the National Health Service. This deliberative task should, in the first instance, be undertaken by the people most concerned – namely 'ordinary' general practitioners.[45]

Though Collings' report proved controversial and may indeed have presented the worst of general practice at the time, it succeeded in bringing general practice to the front pages of the journals and politics. Emerging work identified several issues impacting on general practice – poor infrastructure and work environments, 24-hour service demand, standards of education and care, and very poor remuneration compared to other professions.

In 1951 Hadfield brought together Fraser Rose and John Hunt, both of whom were interested in forming a College of General Practitioners. They started a small steering committee, which subsequently consisted of seven general practitioners and five supportive consultants and which was chaired by Sir Henry Willink, Master of Magdalene College, Cambridge and former Minister of Health. In November 1952 the committee signed the memorandum of articles of association; the College of General Practitioners was legally constituted.[46]

The news of the formation of the College of General Practitioners was enthusiastically embraced by many individual general practitioners. It was well received by the Secretary of the British Medical Association and the Society of Apothecaries, but opposed by the Colleges of Physicians, Surgeons and Obstetricians and Gynaecologists, who wanted general practice to be a joint faculty within their own structures.[47]

The Royal College of General Practitioners grew quickly, having had 1655 members within six weeks,[46] and had developed 22 regional faculties within four years.[47]

Collings returned to Australia and became one of the founding members of the Australian College of General Practitioners, and was one of its first educators.

Box 4.1 lists some of the highlights of the development of general practice, both in terms of the continuing development as a professional organisation around the world and the growth of its professional identity.

BOX 4.1 The development of general practice as a distinct specialty

1946	The *Spence Committee* reported on the very poor remuneration of general practitioners (GPs) and concluded that if GPs were not well paid, recruitment would suffer and only the less able young doctors would enter this branch of medicine, to the detriment of the profession and the public
1947	Foundation of the *American Academy of General Practice*
25 March 1950	Publication in the *Lancet* of the *Collings Report* on General Practice 'General Practice in England Today – a reconnaissance' — key findings: few standards for general practice, no incentives to achieve any, as a result of the national insurance scheme, GPs were stressed and had a low morale. Practice was poorest in proximity to large hospital centres and improved in scope and quality with increasing distance
1950	*Sir Henry Cohen Report*: the status and prestige of the GP should be the equal of colleagues in any and every speciality, and no higher ability, industry or zeal was required for the adequate pursuit of any of them
1951	*Fry* demonstrated the work patterns of GPs: a major component dealt with acute minor ill-health and major disease not requiring hospitalisation, and *Hopkins* showed that a GP refers on average 60 of his 1500 patients per year for a specialist opinion or further management
1951	*Taylor Report*, also commissioned by the Nuffield Provincial Hospital Trust, reported on the best of general practice, concluding that the quality of service depends on the men and women who are actually doing the job; good general practice begins with the good GP
October 1951	*Rose and Hunt*, supported by Hadfield, wrote a letter to the *British Medical Journal* and the *Lancet* to propose the formation of a College of General Practitioners, this was duly opposed by the Royal Colleges of Physicians, Surgeons and Obstetricians and Gynaecologists (who continued to oppose the formation of the other Colleges)
19 November 1952	Foundation of the *College of General Practitioners* as an unincorporated association at 14 Blackfriars Lane, London EC4 (The Society of Apothecaries)
1 January 1953	*Foundation membership* opened: requirement of (i) 20 years in general practice or its equivalent; (ii) 5 years in general practice and giving an undertaking to accept postgraduate instruction for the equivalent of three days a year or five and

	a half days every two years; or (iii) 5 years in general practice and holding a higher postgraduate degree or diploma
21 January 1953	Founding of the *Research Committee*
	Founding of the *Undergraduate Education Committee*
	Founding of the *Postgraduate Education Committee*
1953	*Hadfield Report* on behalf of the British Medical Association: 92% of GPs were adequate or better, 69% left no doubt that patients received what examination was necessary, 75% kept acceptable records; 7% of both young and old GPs needed to revise the methods of diagnosis
1953	The College surveyed universities and found that only Manchester and Edinburgh had a general practice teaching unit, the others were 'planning' to provide some opportunities
June 1954	Foundation of the *College of Family Physicians of Canada*
20 November 1954	First *James Mackenzie Lecture* by WN Pickles, 'Epidemiology in Country Practice'
20 November, 1954	Foundation of the *Examination Committee*
12 October, 1955	Foundation of the *Otago Faculty*
19 November 1955	Interim formation of *Australian* and *New Zealand Councils*
30 October 1956	Foundation of the *Wellington Faculty*
November 1956	Foundation of the *Victoria Faculty*
1956	Foundation of *Kenyan*, *South Ireland*, *Western Australia* and *Canterbury Faculties*
1956	First *Morbidity Survey*
1956	Foundation of the *Dutch College of General Practitioners*
1956	Foundation of the *Indian Academy of General Practice*
19 February 1957	First *New Zealand Council*
5 May 1957	Foundation of the *Tasmania Faculty*
1957	Publication of Michael Balint's book *The Doctor, His Patient and the Illness*[48]
4 February 1958	Foundation of an autonomous *Australian College of General Practitioners*
1960	Foundation of the *Natal* and *Orange Free State Faculties*
13 September 1961	Foundation of the *Northern Transvaal Faculty*
10 March 1962	Foundation of the *Ugandan Faculty*
1963	Publication of *A Guide to Research in General Practice*
1964	Symposium *Art and Science of General Practice*
1 November 1965	First *College Examination*
1966	Foundation of the *German Society of General Practice*
1966	Foundation of the *Austrian Society of General Practice*
17 April 1967	'*Royal*' prefix added to the College title
November 1967	Membership applicants must sit an *examination*
19 May 1968	First *William Pickles Lecture* by P Byrne 'The passing of the "eight" train'

1 July 1968	Foundation of the *South African College of General Practice*
1968	The *Royal Commission into Medical Education* recommended general practice being recognised as a separate discipline requiring its own form of postgraduate training organised by general practitioners
8 February 1969	American Medical Association grant for *Family Medicine* to become the 20th recognised speciality
1969	Publication of *General Practice Teaching of Undergraduates*
1969	16th *James Mackenzie Lecture* by Dr GK Hodgkin entitled 'Behaviour – the community and the GP':

— 'We in our college have gradually gained our confidence and medical recognition by first defining and then preaching that general practice is an academic discipline in its own right. But if the academic status of general practice is to rise, it is necessary to develop an active area of research in a field unique to general practice; to be fully effective this unique field must have wide spread interest and application. It is my thesis that the study of human behaviour provides the general practitioner with just such a unique and interesting field of research.'

1970	Foundation of the *Malta Faculty*
30 June 1971	Foundation the *College of General Practitioners Singapore*
1971	Formation of the *Scottish General Practice Research Unit*
1972	Publication of *The Future General Practitioner – Learning and Teaching*
1972	First Scientific Meeting of the *Departments of General Practice*
1972	*WONCA* (World Organization of National Colleges, Academies and Academic Associations of General Practitioners/Family Physicians) is formed with 18 members
1976	American Academy of Family Physicians introduces *Recertification Examination*
22 July 1977	Foundation of the *Hong Kong College of Family Physicians*
1977	WONCA publication *An International Classification of the Health Problems of Primary Care*
1984	Medical Education Working Party: *mandatory period of general medical education*
1985	Publication of *Quality in General Practice*
1990	Foundation of the *Continuing Medical Education Working Party*
December 1992	Launch of the *Commission on Primary Care*: developing a team approach to patient care through multidisciplinary learning
1992	Foundation of the *Brazilian Society of Family Medicine*

December 1993	Publication of *Portfolio-based Learning in General Practice* (Occasional Paper 63)
1993	Foundation of the *Fiji College of General Practitioners*
June 1994	Publication of *What is Good General Practice?* (Occasional Paper 65)
November 1994	Report *The Development and Implementation of Clinical Guidelines*
February 1995	National Meeting on *Computing in General Practice* Publication of *Influences on Computer Use in General Practice* (Occasional Paper 68)
1995	Canadian College of General Practice introduces *Maintenance of Proficiency Programme*
1997	*Royal College of General Practitioners Bangladesh* and *Royal College of General Practitioners Lebanon* projects
1997	Publication of *Measuring Quality in General Practice* (Occasional Paper 75)
March 1998	Publication of *The Human Side of Medicine*: too much information can discourage a doctor from focusing on the patient as a whole (Occasional Paper 76)
September 1999	Statement on *Revalidation for Clinical General Practice*

CHALLENGES TILL 2020

Many of the original challenges for general practice remain. There is the ongoing need to promote the discipline as one that

> . . . has its own skills and knowledge base that are as important as anything the hospital services might bestow upon it.[47]

The function of the doctor–patient relationship in the consultation was first shown by Hodgkin, a general practitioner and Balint, a psychoanalyst.[48] This work has become one of the leading planks of the discipline. The intrinsic value of the ongoing doctor–patient relationship has been ignored by economists,[49] and has not been sufficiently recognised by many in the discipline. There are some within who view the ongoing doctor–patient relationship as a nostalgic notion that can be replaced by information management tools,[50] despite the overwhelming evidence that the ongoing personal doctor–patient relationship, but not the stable place of care, deliver superior health (and economic) outcomes.[51]

The transformation of general practice, principally kick-started in 1952 by the then Minister of Health in the UK, Iain Macleod, in a speech to the College's Executive Council, still has not been fully implemented. Macleod stressed the desirability of treating as many patients as possible in the community, being better for patients, but also more cost-efficient. This would mean – unequivocally – that the general practitioner should be the leader of a team including midwives, nurses, health visitors, dentists, pharmacists, opticians and so forth, and foster the same kind of team spirit typical of the hospital environment.[47]

SUMMARY POINTS

- The separate distinction of the general practitioner amongst the medical healthcare providers only emerged in the early 1800s.
- Vision, determination, unity and persistence over a period of 140 years finally achieved the foundation of the College of General Practitioners, recognising general practitioners' unique skills and contribution to the health care of the community.
- Governments see general practice as the most desirable place to treat, being best for patients, and being more cost-effective to the community.
- Patients predominantly focus on general practitioners when feeling sick; general practitioners have to rise to the challenge of leading the patients' journey to recovery through a complex healthcare system.

CHAPTER 5

Emerging patterns

Looking back at the history of medicine reveals a number of emerging patterns that still inform the organisation and practice of health care, and in particular primary health care. The very early stages are characterised by the small group recognising *the social importance* to the whole group of caring for the sick and injured (*see* Figure 5.1).

The shaman/medicine man understood the nature of disease, and in particular the patient's understanding of his illness, and developed magic interventions codified in rituals of ceremony and the handing out of medicines (*see* Figure 5.2).

The understanding of disease processes remained largely unclear till the 18th century. Till then medicine was practiced in the Hippocratic tradition and focused on the patient, though the Cnidians unsuccessfully tried to shift the focus of medicine to the disease.

In Roman times health care identified the importance of public and social infrastructure and hygiene – public health was born, though forgotten after the demise of the Roman Empire only to be rediscovered in the middle of the 18th century. Today the public health agenda also address issues such as healthy lifestyle choices, screening

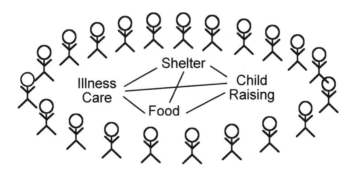

Figure 5.1   The core function of human societies.

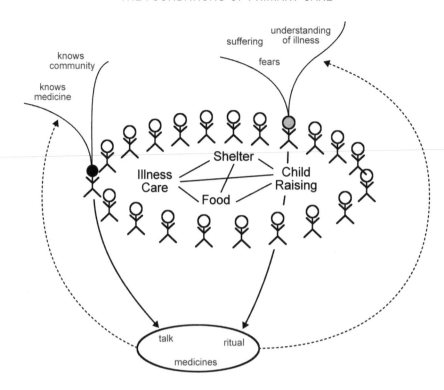

Figure 5.2 The need for medical care.

for preventable diseases, accident prevention, infection control and so forth (*see* Figure 5.3).

In addition to general public health measures we have observed an enormous growth in the knowledge and understanding of the causes and mechanisms of specific diseases. Our ingenuity has led to the development of a multitude of specific technologies for diagnostic and management purposes.

However the science and technology focus has created a layer modifying the inter-actions between doctor and patient. This layer acts like a filter, magnifying the disease aspects, but removing much of the illness experience. The disease focus has led to the fragmentation of medical care, resulting in an ability to cure the patient's diseases without achieving the original aim of medicine – to restore the person to becoming a functioning member of society.

Modern medicine has lost the understanding of the whole, i.e. the person with the illness, in the fragments of his body, organ and cellular parts. Not only science and tech-nology, but also medical education, have shaped a view of medicine as a reductionist enterprise, freeing the discipline from the untidy personal and societal aspects of a patient's life experience. The multifaceted nature of disease and illness was familiar to our predecessors – the shamen/medicine men, Hippocrates, Osler, Feinstein – who all addressed the complexities of the patient's lifeworld into their treatments (*see* Figure 5.4).

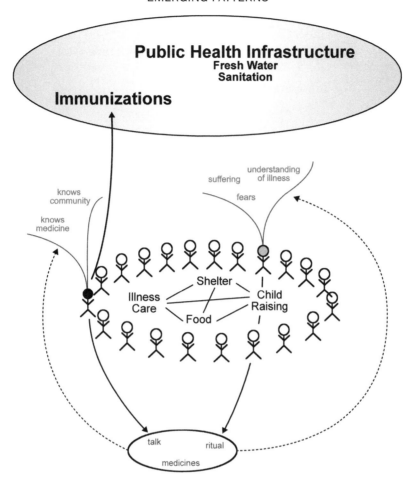

Figure 5.3 Health is also dependent upon public health measures.

FURTHER READING

Diffin J. *History of Medicine: a scandalously short introduction.* University of Toronto Press, 1999.

REFERENCES

1 Tiger L and Fox R. *The Imperial Animal.* New York: Holt, Rinehart and Winston, 1971.

2 May W. *The Physician's Covenant: images of the healer in medical ethics.* Philadelphia: The Westminster Press, 1983.

3 *The Macquarie Dictionary* (2e). Sydney: The Macquarie Library Pty, 1988.

4 Rosenberg C. Disease in history: frames and framers. *Milbank Quarterly.* 1989; **67**(Suppl 1): 1–15.

5 McCormick J. The contribution of science to medicine. *Perspectives in Biology and Medicine.* 1993; **36**: 315–22.

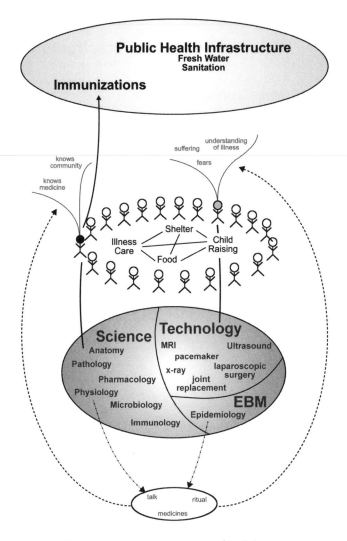

Figure 5.4 The impact of modern understanding on the task of medicine.

6 Capra F. *The Turning Point: science, society and the rising culture.* Toronto: Batman Books, 1983.

7 Carr I. *The Far Beginnings – A Brief History of Medicine.* www.umanitoba.ca/faculties/ medicine/history/histories/briefhis.html (accessed 30 June 2006).

8 Hammurabi KoB. *The Oldest Code of Laws in the World.* www.gutenberg.org/files/17150/17150-h/17150-h.htm (accessed 30 June 2006).

9 *A History of Medicine.* www.historylearningsite.co.uk\history_of_medicine.htm (accessed 30 June 2006).

10 Eliot TS. The Rock. In: T S Eliot. *Complete Poems and Plays: 1909–1950.* London: Harcourt, 1952. p.48.

11 Centre for the Evaluation of Risks to Human Reproduction (CERHR). *Thalidomide.* CERHR, 2005. http://cerhr.niehs.nih.gov/common/thalidomide.html (accessed 30 June 2006)

12 Persaud T. Hippocrates on the Web. History of Medicine, Faculty of Medicine, University of Manitoba. *Human Anatomy: early history.* www.umanitoba.ca/faculties/medicine/units/history/notes/anatomy/ (accessed 30 June 2006).

13 McKeown T. *The Modern Rise of Population.* London: Edward Arnold, 1976.

14 Sedivy R. Rokitansky und die Wiener Medizinische Schule. Von der Naturphilosophie zur Naturwissenschaft. *Wiener Medizinische Wochenschrift.* 2004; **154**: 443–53.

15 Sedivy R. 200 Jahre Rokitansky – sein Vermächtnis für die heutige Pathologie. *Wiener Klinische Wochenschrift.* 2004; **116**: 779–87.

16 Morabia A. A new look at the relation of epidemiology and bacteriology at the turn of the 20th century. *Sozial und Präventivmedizin.* 2001; **46**: 352–3.

17 Vandenbroucke J. Changing images of John Snow in the history of epidemiology. *Sozial und Präventivmedizin.* 2001; **46**: 288–93.

18 Vineis P. Causality in epidemiology. *Sozial und Präventivmedizin.* 2003; **48**: 80–7.

19 Doll R and Hill A. Smoking and carcinoma of the lung. Preliminary report. *British Medical Journal.* 1950; **II**(4682): 739–48.

20 Richmond C. Sir Richard Doll. *British Medical Journal.* 2005; **331**: 295. http://bmj.bmjjournals.com/cgi/content/full/331/7511/295/DC1 (accessed 30 June 2006).

21 Framingham Heart Study. www.nhlbi.nih.gov/about/framingham/ (accessed 30 June 2006).

22 Bean B. *Sir William Osler Aphorisms* (2e). Springfield, Illinois, USA: Charles C Thomas, 1961.

23 University of Virginia. *Antiqua Medicina. From Homer to Vesalius.* www.healthsystem.virginia.edu/internet/library/historical/artifacts/antiqua/ (accessed 30 June 2006).

24 Siraisi NG. Medicine and the Renaissance world of learning. *Bulletin of History in Medicine.* 2004; **78**: 1–36.

25 Flexner A. *Medical Education in the United States and Canada. A Report to the Carnegie Foundation for the Advancement of Teaching.* New York: Carnegie Foundation, 1910.

26 Dornan T. Osler, Flexner, apprenticeship and 'the new medical education'. *Journal of the Royal Society of Medicine.* 2005; **98**: 91–5.

27 Hiatt M and Stockton C. The impact of the Flexner Report on the fate of medical schools in North America after 1909. *Journal of the American Physicians and Surgeons* 2003; **8**: 37–40.

28 McWhinney I. Family medicine in perspective. *New England Journal of Medicine.* 1975; **293**: 176–81.

29 McWhinney I. Medical knowledge and the rise of technology. *Journal of Medicine and Philosophy.* 1978; **3**: 293–304.

30 Croockshank F. The theory of diagnosis. Part I. *Lancet* 1926; **6 November**: 939–42.

31 Flexner A. *Universities, American, English and German.* New York: Oxford University Press, 1930.

32 McWhinney I. The importance of being different. William Pickles Lecture 1996. *British Journal of General Practice.* 1996; **46**: 433–6.

33 Hart J. The world turned upside down: proposals for community-based undergraduate medical education. *British Journal of General Practice.* 1985; **35**: 63–8.

34 Kaufman A, Klepper D, Obenshain S *et al.* Undergraduate medical education for primary care: a case study in New Mexico. *The Southern Medical Journal.* 1982; **75**: 1110–17.

35 Kaufman A, Mennin S, Waterman R *et al.* The New Mexico experiment: educational innovation and institutional change. *Academic Medicine.* 1989; **64**: 285–94.

36 Mirghani O, El Amin E, Ali M, Osman H and Hamad B. A combined course of primary health care practice and family medicine at the University of Gezira. *Medical Education.* 1988; **22**: 314–16.

37 Brazeau N, Potts M and Hickner J. The Upper Peninsula Program: a successful model for increasing primary care physicians in rural areas. *Family Medicine.* 1990; **22**: 350–5.

38 Worley P, Silagy C, Prideaux D, Newble D and Jones A. The parallel rural community curriculum: an integrated clinical curriculum based in rural general practice. *Medical Education.* 2000; **34**: 558–65.

39 Sturmberg J, Reid A and Khadra M. Community based medical education in a rural area: a new direction in undergraduate training. *Australian Journal of Rural Health.* 2001; **9**(Suppl 1): S14–S18.

40 Baron R. An introduction to medical phenomenology: I can't hear you while I'm listening. *Annals of Internal Medicine.* 1985; **103**: 606–11.

41 Sturmberg J, Reid A, Thacker J and Chamberlain C. A community based, patient-centred, longitudinal medical curriculum. *Rural and Remote Health (online)* 2003; **3**(no. 210). http://rrh.deakin.edu.au/articles/subviewnew.asp?ArticleID=210 (accessed 30 June 2006).

42 Beairsto B. Learning that lasts. Changing our minds – literally! Ministry of Education and SDCBC webcast, 4 May 2005. www.insinc.com\ministryofeducation\20050504\presentation-archive.html (accessed 30 June 2006).

43 University of New South Wales. *Expectations for Level of Achievement of the Graduate Capabilities in Each Phase of the Curriculum.* www.med.unsw.edu.au/medweb.nsf/resources/GraduateCapabilities/$file/GraduateCapabilities.pdf (accessed 30 June 2006).

44 Loudon S. The origin of the general practitioner. *Journal of the Royal College of General Practitioners.* 1983; **33**: 13–18.

45 Collings J. General practice in England today – a reconnaissance? *Lancet.* 1950; **i**: 555–85.

46 Tait I. *The History of the RCGP.* www.rcgp.org.uk/history/histories/historyessay/index.asp (accessed 30 June 2006).

47 *Rethinking the National Health Service.* www.nhshistory.net/1948–1957.htm (accessed 30 June 2006).

48 Balint M. *The Doctor, His Patient and the Illness* (2e). Edinburgh, London, Melbourne and New York: Churchill Livingstone, 1986.

49 Hart J. Expectations of health care: promoted, managed or shared? *Health Expectations.* 1998; **1**: 3–13.

50 Fleming D. Continuity of care: a concept revisited. *European Journal of General Practice.* 2000; **6**: 140–5.

51 Saultz JW and Lochner J. Interpersonal continuity of care and care outcomes: a critical review. *Annals of Family Medicine.* 2005; **3**: 159–66.

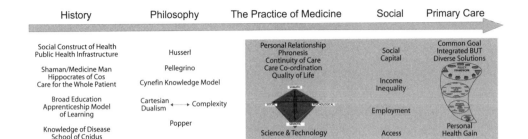

History	Philosophy	The Practice of Medicine	Social	Primary Care

Social Construct of Health
Public Health Infrastructure

Shaman/Medicine Man
Hippocrates of Cos
Care for the Whole Patient

Broad Education
Apprenticeship Model
of Learning

Knowledge of Disease
School of Cnidus

Husserl

Pellegrino

Cynefin Knowledge Model

Cartesian ←→ Complexity
Dualism

Popper

Personal Relationship
Phronesis
Continuity of Care
Care Co-ordination
Quality of Life

Science & Technology

Social
Capital

Income
Inequality

Employment

Access

Common Goal
Integrated BUT
Diverse Solutions

Personal
Health Gain

SECTION 2

Philosophical perspective of medicine: search for the meaning of health and illness

The philosopher should begin with medicine; the physician should end with philosophy.

Aristotle

The best physician is also a philosopher.

Galen of Pergamum

It would be palpably unwise to attempt to make every physician a philosopher, in Galen's or Plato's sense. But every physician, since he is involved with values, concepts, and ideas of medicine, must have some philosophical *sense*.

Pellegrino and Thomasma[1]

Philosophy determines the way we explain ourselves and the world around us. This section aims to highlight some of the important issues of the medical and scientific philosophies that have shaped medical practice and research, as well as introduce the emerging view of understanding health and health care through systems and complexity thinking.

It is not possible, and indeed would be pretentious, to offer either an in-depth, complete or definite view. However, I hope that readers will gain a feel for the traditional thoughts that have shaped medicine, and discover how these still shape the enquiry and delivery of health care.

The first chapter in this section introduces some of the philosophical traditions of medicine all of which have one thing in common – health is constructed as a balanced state, and illness as a disruption of this balance. Medical care aims to restore the balance and the health of the patient by making sense out of the illness experience. While universal, this concept is time and culture sensitive, i.e. for patients from different backgrounds the same illness may provide a different experience and/or meaning. As a discipline, medicine is characterised by its clinical interaction in the consultation.

The second chapter explores some of the issues underpinning science and knowledge generation. The first part traces the rise of the natural sciences which are grounded in Descartes' approach of deductive reasoning and its associated determinism, which in turn have given rise to the mechanistic world view of the Newtonian paradigm. The methods of science are based on observation of natural phenomena; however, as Popper has argued, observations are never objective since observations always require a focus. The successes of science and technology in medicine are undeniable; the downside though has been the neglect of the person. The second part explores the concept of knowledge and knowing, concluding that there are many different ways of knowing, and that much of our knowledge is not readily transferable. The Cynefin framework offers the means of understanding and managing our knowledge more effectively.

Chapter 8 introduces systems and complexity thinking. The mechanistic world view is no longer sustainable as we start to rediscover that the real world is one large interconnected whole.

The impact of the above on medicine are succinctly summarised by Pellegrino and Thomasma:

> Medicine clearly is a domain of activity which is distinctive and distinguishable as science, art, and praxis . . . It is precisely the clinical encounter that constitutes the singular ordering concept which distinguishes medicine from the sciences and which is the ground for the logic, the epistemology, and the metaphysics of medical practice.[1]

CHAPTER 6

Some philosophical
fragments on medicine

Medicine is as fundamental as any human endeavor for the revelation
of what it means to be human. As such, it offers a fruitful source for
philosophical reflection. Medicine, in turn, needs philosophy. Critical
reflection on the 'style' and content of medicine will aid its own self-
understanding and the patient's self-understanding as well.

Pellegrino and Thomasma[1]

Much of the philosophy of medicine is pragmatic and linked to the historical and social
role of the physician. As briefly described in Chapter 1, medicine was based on a social
need, the need to care for ill or injured members to secure the survival of the whole
group. Caring for the ill soon became a formalised role – the group entrusted the caring
for the sick into the shaman/medicine man, and in return granted him the privilege of
being exempted from hunting. Besides healing the sick, he was responsible for directing
communal sacrifice and escorting the dead to another world.

The origins of medicine were deeply embedded in the fabric of society and clearly
holistic in nature, embracing physical as well as spiritual needs, for both the patient and
the community at large.

Not surprisingly then, medicine and philosophy were closely linked from antiquity
to the Middle Ages, and medical education was truly interdisciplinary involving the
arts, literature, politics, astrology, and to a large extent religion.[1] The initial superstitious
nature of disease was rejected by Hippocrates who for the first time observed that illness
has natural causes and cures – the beginning of the era of 'scientific medicine'.

The doctor always had a privileged position in society coupled with a set of expected
behaviours and duties. These have been enshrined in the Hippocratic Oath which is

neither ethically neutral nor value free, and thus describes a practice that inseparably links medical and ethical concerns.[2]

BOX 6.1 The Hippocratic Oath

I swear by Apollo the physician, and Aesculapius, and Hygieia, and Panacea, and all the gods and goddesses that, according to my ability and judgement, I will keep this Oath and this stipulation:

To reckon him who taught me this Art equally dear to me as my parents, to share my substance with him and relieve his necessities if required; to look upon his offspring in the same footing as my own brothers, and to teach them this Art, if they shall wish to learn it, without fee or stipulation, and that by precept, lecture, and every other mode of instruction, I will impart a knowledge of the Art to my own sons and those of my teachers, and to disciples bound by a stipulation and oath according to the law of medicine, but to none others.

I will follow that system of regimen which, according to my ability and judgement, I consider for the benefit of my patients, and abstain from whatever is deleterious and mischievous. I will give no deadly medicine to any one if asked, nor suggest any such counsel; and in like manner I will not give a woman a pessary to produce abortion.

With purity and with holiness I will pass my life and practise my Art. I will not cut persons labouring under the stone, but will leave this to be done by men who are practitioners of this work. Into whatever houses I enter I will go into them for the benefit of the sick and will abstain from every voluntary act of mischief and corruption; and further from the seduction of females or males, of freemen and slaves.

Whatever, in connection with my professional practice, or not in connection with it, I may see or hear in the lives of men which ought not to be spoken of abroad I will not divulge, as reckoning that all such should be kept secret.

While I continue to keep this Oath unviolated may it be granted to me to enjoy life and the practice of the Art, respected by all men, in all times! But should I trespass and violate this Oath, may the reverse be my lot!

HEALTH AND ILLNESS: INTERDEPENDENT RELATIVE STATES

Alcmaeon of Croton (circa 535–unknown BC) was the first physician to postulate health as a balance between the powers of the body fluids – heat and cold, moisture and dryness, bitterness and sweetness. If one fluid dominated over the other, illness developed.

Based on these ideas, Hippocrates of Cos (460–380 BC) developed the Theory of the Four Humours (*see* Figure 6.1), which, with further refinements by Galen of Pergamum (131–200 AD), became the principle guidelines for diagnosing and treating patients well into the 18th century (*see* Tables 6.1 and 6.2).

The notion of health and illness being a balanced state is deeply anchored in the explanatory models of health and disease in many cultural traditions.[1] Hence the philosophical ideas underlying health and disease are, not surprisingly, similar

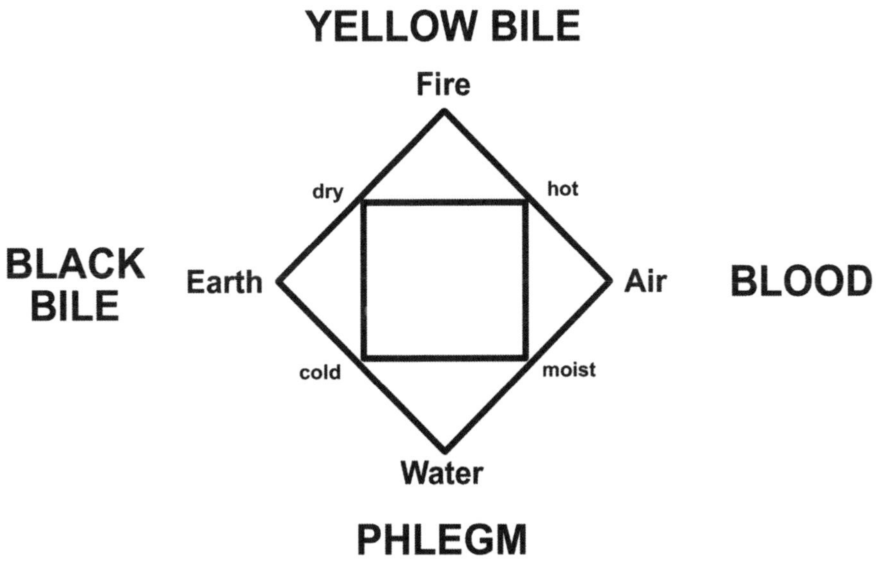

YELLOW BILE

BLACK BILE

BLOOD

PHLEGM

Figure 6.1 Hippocratic Theory of the Four Humours.

incorporating physical, environmental and spiritual components (*see* Table 6.3). All balance models acknowledge the complex interactions between the different aspects of human existence, and treatments accordingly embrace a variety of methods to restore the imbalances of the physical, environmental and spiritual dimensions.

TABLE 6.1 Hippocratic diagnosis and treatment[3]

SYMPTOM	DIAGNOSIS	TREATMENT
Patient is feverish, dry	Excess yellow bile	Cold baths
Patient is feverish, sweating, and flushed	Excess of blood	Bleeding
Patient is cool, dry, lethargic	Excess black bile	Build up blood, feed patient red meat, red wine

Chapter 11 will expand on the balance notion of health, and Chapter 12 will examine its impact on contemporary medicine in greater detail. At this point it should be emphasised again that

> . . . the archaic roots of medicine . . . [are] buried under the biomedical science facade of modern health care . . . [and that] we really know [little] about the most central function of clinical care.[4] (p. 312)

It should also not be surprising that the traditional models of health care are alive and well, and that patients who feel 'let down' by modern medicine return to the 'roots of medical care', typically practised by practitioners commonly classed as 'alternative'.

TABLE 6.2 The Ancient Theory of the Four Humours and their influence on medicine (adapted from: Wikipedia 2006, http://en.wikipedia.org/wiki/The_four_humours)

DATE	ORIGINATOR	DESCRIPTIONS			
~400 BC	Hippocrates' four humours	Yellow bile	Black bile	Phlegm	Blood
	Season	Summer	Autumn	Winter	Spring
	Element	Fire	Earth	Water	Air
	Organ	Liver	Brain/lungs	Gall bladder	Spleen
	Characteristics	Dry and hot	Dry and cold	Wet and cold	Wet and hot
		Easily angered, bad tempered	Despondent, sleepless, irritable	Calm, unemotional	Courageous, hopeful, amorous
~325 BC	Aristotle's four sources of happiness	Hedone (sensuous pleasure)	Propraitari (acquiring assets)	Ethikos (moral virtue)	Dialogike (logical investigation)
~190 AD	Galen's four temperaments	Choleric	Melancholic	Phlegmatic	Sanguine
~1550	Paracelsus' four totem spirits	Changeable salamanders	Industrious gnomes	Inspired nymphs	Curious sylphs
~1905	Adicke's four world views	Innovative	Traditional	Doctrinaire	Sceptical
~1914	Spränger's four value attitudes	Artistic	Economic	Religious	Theoretic
~1920	Kretchmer's four character styles	Hypomanic	Depressive	Hyperaesthetic	Anaesthetic
~1947	Erich Fromm's four orientations	Exploitative	Hoarding	Receptive	Marketing
~1958	Myers' cognitive function types	SP – sensory perception	SI – sensory judgement	NF – intuitive feeling	NT – intuitive thinking
~1978	Keirsey's four temperaments	Artisan	Guardian	Idealist	Rational

TABLE 6.3 Traditions and Practice of Medicine (Compiled from Stoyan-Rosenzweig N. *Balancing the Humors: healing traditions and medical practice in world medicine*[3])

TRADITION	PRINCIPLES OF HEALTH MODEL	ILLNESS: CAUSES AND EFFECTS	RESTORATION OF HEALTH
Hippocratic	Balance of humours: • universe: paired opposite forces • four humours/elements • humours are observed during illness	Imbalance of humours: • habits: poor hygiene, diet, lack of or excessive activity • unhealthy surroundings • time of the year • constitution/temperament	Treatments: • remove excess • build up humour • diet, exercise, bleeding, purging, cathartic, blistering, emetic, surgery, bandage • individual treatment
Chinese	Balance of yin yang: • body represents the microcosm of the universe and its processes • Qi – the life energy – flows through the body • cycling of yin and yang forces five elements – wood, fire, earth, metal, water • yin and yang are not polar opposites, one is not exclusive of the other, both are needed to achieve balance and go though a regular cycle • some organs are dominated by yin (solid organs), others by yang (hollow organs)	Bodies out of balance: • yin-yang imbalance leads to improper movement of chi in channels • external pathogens – cold, heat, wind, moisture, dryness, internal heat • internal upset – emotions, foods • imbalance of a particular element or phase – people ruled by a particular element are more likely to have an imbalance of that element	Treatments: • five methods of treatment – living in harmony with nature; treatment of bowels, viscera, blood and breath; control of diet; drugs; acupuncture/moxibustion • surgery is traditionally not important • herbal meditation, Tai Chi, Chi gong and other martial arts
Ayurvedic	Balance of the three dosas: kapha, pitta, vatta • body represents microcosm of universe • individual is a unique combination of his dosas	Bodies out of balance: • imbalance of particular dosa has specific effects on part of body • unbalanced blood • external toxins and pathogens, spirits, factors within the body	Treatments: • vegetable-based medicine • diet – issues of combining or not combining certain foods • extensive surgery – may be a separate tradition • meditation – yoga • bleeding • gems, colours
Tibetan	Balance of: • mind and body • spiritual, magic and rational • three poisons linked to humours	Bodies out of balance: • ultimately caused by ignorance • poisons can throw humours out of balance • external cause of imbalance – climate, demons/spirits, diet, behaviour • nature of disease • disorders of humours • karmic disorder	Treatments: • correct imbalance • spiritual transformation • treat the whole person – the illness and the person • diet, beverages, herbal medicines • moxibustion • bloodletting

MEDICINE AND THE 'COMMON GOOD'

Socrates (470–399 BC) saw an important link between the virtuous standing of a person and the standing of his physical health. He compared the moral philosopher's approach to achieve restoration of a person's virtues with that of the doctor's attempt to achieve restoration of a person's physical health.

Socrates points out that both must be skilled in their craft, they must: (1) be able to explain their own procedures; (2) know the real nature of their task; and (3) serve the human good.[2] Knowing one's craft is more than knowing its content, and more than the knowledge one gains from observation. True craft reflects the feel of one's own skilled performance.

These attributes of *skill and purpose* are still relevant for today's physicians. In his 2001 paper Mark Moes highlights 10 parallel ideas between Socrates' understanding of health and illness, and virtue and vice.[2] Socrates identified these analogies between the moral philosopher and the doctor:

> Moral vice, on the contrary, like disease, is an inward condition that does limit or prevent the actualization and operation of uniquely human activities.

> . . . 'a fit body doesn't by its own virtue make the soul good, but instead the opposite is true – a good soul by its own virtue make the body as good as possible.' Though physical health can be enhanced by moral virtue, physical health does not suffice to make one virtuous.

> . . . that the spiritual capacity of humans means that good physical health is not only not sufficient for worthy living, but also not even altogether necessary. A person suffering simultaneously from ulcers, chronic emphysema, psoriasis, tumors, a limp, and heart problems might nevertheless live a vibrant human life filled with intellectual activity and with loving relationships . . .

> On Socrates' account, health is a natural standard or norm, the well-working of a person as a whole . . .

> . . . just as there are forms of disease whose symptoms, courses, and causes are common knowledge to doctors, so there are forms of vice whose symptoms, courses and causes are common knowledge to the wise . . .

> . . . the virtuous person is more-or-less invulnerable to strong temptations to exchange higher for lesser values or to give in to powerful corruptive influences in his social, cultural, and spiritual environment, just as the healthy body is highly resistant to potentially powerful corruptive influences from the bodily environment.

> . . . both health and virtue are conditions that can be apparently but not really present.

> . . . one must be willing to commit oneself to a program of physical regimen if one wishes to develop physically.

> . . . just as one's bodily health affects the way one reacts to foods and other stimuli, so the condition of one's soul influences the way in which one is affected by thoughts, suggestions, and perceptions.

The human body seems to possess powers of self-construction, self-maintenance, self-repair, and self-transformation. Among other things, it possesses an immune system. Good doctors recognize the point at which to step in and to help a natural urge to self-healing already at work within the patient.[2]

Socrates also explored the doctor–patient relationship, highlighting that patients are able to co-operate with their doctor, and can accept some responsibility for their condition. Socrates views doctors neither as mere servants of their patients' wishes, nor as despotic masters. In a well-functioning doctor–patient relationship, both will be able to recognise when and how to activate the patient's self-healing properties.

THE EMPHASIS OF MEDICINE: DISEASE OR ILLNESS, CURE OR CARE

What should be the emphasis of medicine? The question itself is an old one, and to all intents and purposes has not yet been resolved. The answer to this question may well be the lynchpin to the survival of medicine as we know it.

Hippocrates once more may provide some insights:

Disease is not caused by demons or capricious deities but rather by natural forces that obey natural laws. Hence, therapeutic procedures can be developed on a rational basis. These procedures include the use of regimens, drugs and surgical techniques designed to correct the ill effects of natural forces.

The well-being of man is under the influence of the environment, including in particular air, water, places and the various regimens. The understanding of the effect of the environment on man is the fundamental basis of the physician's art.

Health is the expression of a harmonious balance between the various components of man's nature (the four humours that control all human activities) and the environment and ways of life. Whatever happens in the mind influences the body and vice versa. In fact, mind and body cannot be considered independently one from the other.

Health means a healthy mind in a healthy body, and can be achieved only by governing daily life in accordance with natural laws, which ensures equilibrium between the different forces of the organism and those of the environment.

Medicine is an ethical profession and implies an attitude of reverence for the human condition.

As far back as the 5th century BC the schools of Cnid and Cos debated what is of importance to medical practice – to describe and cure diseases, or to describe the illness and care for the patient with the aim of *restoring his wholeness*. The acceptance of the Cartesian dualism, i.e. the split of the mind from the body, in the 17th century reignited the difference in approach to the practice of medicine, and challenged the prevailing Hippocratic view.

The effects of the Cartesian split prevail – Cartesianism through its reductionist approaches being a source of great strength and at the same time its greatest deficiency.[1] They have become more obvious in our times of scientific and technological development, and the increasing emphasis on evidence and evidence-based medicine, and in fact are the dominant force in contemporary Western medicine. Ducan examined the question of *what* matters to medicine in his 1984 address to the Royal Society of Medicine entitled 'Caring or Curing: conflicts of choice'.[5] He reached the conclusion that in light of the limited benefit of curative approaches we must concern ourselves much more with the quality of life issues affecting our patients, jointly define the objectives of management, and revise them as time progresses.

MEDICINE AND THE LIFEWORLD

The history of medicine is indeed the history of people's individual experience of problems and the way they, their communities and their healers have dealt with them. Historically, explanations and treatments belong together – initially they were magico-religious, today they are biopsychosocial.[1,6]

There is no arguing about the insights and benefits gained from science for modern medicine. However being sick and getting better (or for that matter dying) is a personal experience that occurs in the real lifeworld of the patient. Illness and the clinical relationship are experienced in the context of the patient's real lifeworld of the here and now, and in the cultural context of society, of which science is but one part.

This lifeworld concept goes back to the German philosopher Edmund Husserl (1859–1938). He recognised that no phenomenon exists *per se*, that every phenomenon is only recognisable through its experience. Each experience provides us with *meaning*, and has a *value* attached to it. No experience is value free. In addition the lifeworld experience has a social dimension, it occurs in a community rooted in time.[1] Different communities and different times have their unique lifeworld experiences, and thus provide different *meaning* to their experiences. Most readers would be able to relate to this in the context of dealing with indigenous, immigrant or refugee patients. The cross-cultural differences of the illness experience have been explored in great detail by Kleinman.[7]

The following excerpts from Pellegrino and Thomasma's 1981 book *A Philosophical Basis of Medical Practice. Towards a philosophy and ethic of the healing professions*[1] outline some of the challenges for medicine as a discipline, and for doctors as care providers in their interactions with the real lifeworld of all their patients.

> Professionals and laymen are distinguished by their degree of involvement in either world: that of theory or that of everyday experience. Both are interrelated. One cannot presume that the ability to name a disorder experienced in the everyday world automatically means that one 'knows' more about the disorder than the patient. The patient has a richer, more personal knowledge of the disorder because it is happening to him or her. The physician only has a more theoretical knowledge of the disorder due to training. The relationship between theory and practice means that the personal situation of the patient must be taken into account in any theoretical attempt to explain and dislodge the disease.

In recent years Chester Burns and Alasdair MacIntyre have both analyzed the medical enterprise historically in search of norms and an ethics for modern medicine. Both have highlighted the relationship of the profession to canons and norms of the everyday world. With the dissolution of absolute norms, and in the face of the moral pluralism of our times, medicine is left normless. It is a sea with ancient life preservers, so to speak. Theory is left behind by the changing lifeworld. As James says at the end of his *Varieties of Religious Experience*, 'Assuredly the real world is of a different temperament—more intricately built than science allows.'

The idea of a lifeworld, or world of practical experience, is important for a philosophy of medicine because medicine is a practical discipline, a discipline of experience in which much theory is theory about practice. Medicine must make correct decisions on behalf of patients. In addition, medicine proceeds by analogical thinking. In medicine, a disease is identified through a syndrome of patterns analogous with each other. And as Buchanan observes, 'you never get an abstraction out of this.' Theory in medicine is theory about the world of everyday reality, about fundamental human values played out in daily life. Thus, in medicine, reflective reasoning operates along with ordinary, unreflective knowledge.[1]

HOW TO DEFINE MEDICINE

There are no agreed definitions of what constitutes medicine, and the views shared are those articulated by Pellegrino and Thomasma.[1] The basis of medicine is characterised by its *practice* – the interactions between the doctor and the patient in the clinical event.

> The special character of the relationship between physician and patient, the goals of that relationship, and the ways in which they are affected in the moment of clinical decision set medicine apart from all other related activities, particularly the other helping professions.[1]

The conceptions of medicine, health and disease are related, and receive their meaning through the clinical interaction. Health and disease are evaluative concepts, i.e. their meaning includes the values of patients, society and culture. The aim of the medical interaction is to restore the patient's wellbeing, and the clinical interaction itself is characterised by

> . . . four modes – responsibility, trust, decision orientation, and etiology – [and] are the essential ingredients of a medical event. All are tied together and represent categories of importance to the clinical relationship.

> . . . Medicine is the cognitive art of applying science and persuasion through a complex human interaction in which a mutually satisfactory state of well-being is sought, and in which the uniqueness of values and disease, and the kind of institution in which care is delivered, determine the nature of the judgments made.

Two personal intentions at least are needed to form a clinical interaction, both with a curative intent, one to seek help and the other to extend it. The link between intentions is the special character of the event. Since it is cognitive (diagnosis), predictive (prognosis), operative (therapeutic), affective (friendship or trust), and cultural (beliefs about man, nature, and society), the clinical interaction establishes medicine as a tekné iatrikê, a technique of healing. Tekné here means a knowledge of how to act according to what is the case and why it is the case.[1]

The importance of these principles will become more apparent in the next sections in relation to our understanding of disease, illness and health; the role of the doctor in society; and the conception of the healthcare system at large.

SUMMARY POINTS

- About 500 BC, Alcmaeon of Croton postulated the concept of health being a balance, and illness an imbalance of the body fluids, a concept found in virtually all medical traditions.
- Based on Alcmaeon's concept, Hippocrates developed the Theory of the Four Humours which remained the framework for medical thinking and practice well into the 18th century.
- Health and illness are relative rather than discrete absolute states.
- Socrates viewed good physical health as not only not sufficient for worthy living, but also not even altogether necessary for a vibrant human life filled with intellectual activity and with loving relationships, thereby defining *health* as a personal and experiential concept.
- A well-functioning doctor–patient relationship activates the patient's self-healing properties.
- The historical aim of medicine, encapsulated as the Hippocratic tradition of medicine, is to diagnose the *patient's illness* and *restore his wholeness*.
- The 17th century acceptance of the Cartesian dualism conceptualised the human body in the man-machine metaphor, the basis for the reductionist approach, and the foundation of the prevailing disease focus in medicine.
- The late 19th century re-introduced the basic concepts of health being a contextual experience, and that healing occurs by making sense of the illness experience.
- The basis of medicine is its *practice*, i.e. it is defined by the interaction between doctor and patient in the clinical encounter.
- Health and disease are value-laden concepts whose understanding depends on the patients, society and culture.

CHAPTER 7

Philosophical fragments on science

The term 'science' or 'scientific' is often used in the press and the professional literature and seems to imply that what is stated is especially meritorious or reliable. This
conjecture raises many questions. What do we really mean by 'science'? How does
'science' work? What is 'science' telling us? What is the basis for the implied authority
of 'science'?

Two people were principally responsible for the development of modern science.
Francis Bacon (1561–1626) introduced the inductive method to gaining new knowledge
based on experiments. René Descartes (1596–1659) rejected Bacon's notion and
postulated the deductive method to establishing the truth based on first principles/laws.
His viewpoint prevailed and became the basis for and successes of almost all scientific
work for the next 400 years.

Descartes also introduced the machine metaphor to describe the functioning of
the body, and set the body apart from the mind. (In retrospect this may have been a
clever political move to on the one hand allow *the new way of enquiry* to proceed and
on the other to satisfy the orthodoxy of the Roman Church, which was vehemently
opposed to and threatened by the discoveries of scientists like Galileo and Copernicus.)
This concept is known as the Cartesian dualism, and has survived into our times.
The machine metaphor embodies the notion that the body can be reduced into its
distinctive parts without losing its overall 'machine-like' character. It follows that fully
understanding the parts imparts complete knowledge about the whole body (machine)
– the *deductive method* aims to *determine outcomes*, and is the rationale for reductionist
thinking.

Isaac Newton (1643–1727) embraced Descartes' views. They were fundamental to
his thinking and the development of the foundations of modern science.[8]

The logic behind Newtonian science is easy to formulate . . . Its best known principle, which was formulated by the philosopher-scientist Descartes well before Newton, is that of analysis or reductionism: to understand any complex phenomenon, you need to take it apart, i.e. reduce it to its individual components. If these are still complex, you need to take your analysis one step further, and look at their components.[8]

Newton's foundational work culminated in the 1687 publication of his book *The Principia or Mathematical Principles of Natural Philosophy*. In it he defined the concepts of absolute time and absolute space, mass, momentum and gravitation, leading to his three laws of motion. These allowed him to reduce phenomena by the application of general principles, a method which proved to be highly productive, and which shaped the *mechanistic* views and the methods of the 'scientific' world into our times – the Newtonian paradigm.

SCIENCE AND TRUTH

Socrates was executed not for saying what things were or should be, but for seeking practical indications of where some reasonable approximation of truth might be. He was executed not for his megalomania or grandiose propositions or certitudes, but for stubbornly doubting the absolute truths of others.

John Ralston Saul – The Unconscious Civilisation[9]

The chief cause of poverty in science is imaginary wealth. The chief aim of science is not to open a door to infinite wisdom, but to set a limit to infinite error.

Berthold Brecht – The Life of Galileo[10]

'Scientific' research is widely seen as providing 'truth' about the natural world. The 'scientific' process starts with the generation of a hypothesis and is followed by the design of experiments and the rigorous observation of their outcomes. Results that support the hypothesis are seen as proof, and hence are believed to be true. However truth is rather elusive. Socrates is but one of many who paid with their life for doubting 'absolute truths'.

Karl Popper (1902–1994) in his famous paper *Science: conjectures and refutations* examined three basic assumptions underpinning scientific enterprise – the nature of hypothesis generation, the status of observations, and the notion that falsifiability is the ultimate test of any good theory.[11]

Popper argued against the inductive method of hypothesis generation. Rather than making repetitive observations and looking for similarities that allow us to generate rules, we jump to conclusions, look for observations that support our conclusion, or otherwise disregard them. We use a method of trial and error – conjectures and refutations. He concluded:

that scientific theories were not the digest of observations, but that they were inventions – conjectures boldly put forward for trial, to be eliminated if they clashed with observations; with observations which were rarely accidental but as a rule undertaken with the definite intention of testing a theory by obtaining, if possible, a decisive refutation.[11]

OBSERVATIONS

Observations have been regarded as the means to test all scientific theory. However the doctrine of '*seeing is believing*' has rarely been examined, despite doubts being raised over a long period of time. To demonstrate the unsustainability of the proposition Popper started a 1927 lecture with the instructions:

> Take pencil and paper; carefully observe, and write down what you have observed! They asked, of course, what I wanted them to observe. Clearly the instruction, 'Observe!' is absurd.[11]

Observations, rather than being objective, as has been and still is widely believed, are

> . . . always selective. [Observation] needs a chosen object, a definite task, an interest, a point of view, a problem.[11]

VERIFICATION AND FALSIFICATION

And finally Popper showed that a good scientific theory must be open to refutation or falsifiability. He concluded that:

1   It is easy to obtain confirmations, or verifications, for merely every theory – if we look for confirmations.

2   Confirmations should count only if they are the result of risky predictions; that is to say, if, unenlightened by the theory in question, we should have expected an event which was incompatible with the theory – an event which would have refuted the theory.

3   A theory which is not refutable by any conceivable event is non-scientific. Irrefutability is not a virtue of a theory (as people often think) but a vice.

4   Every genuine test of a theory is an attempt to falsify it, or to refute it. Testability is falsifiability; but there are degrees of testability: some theories are more testable, more exposed to refutation, than others; they take, as it were, greater risks.

5   Confirming evidence should not count except when it is the result of a genuine test of the theory; and this means that it can be presented as a serious but unsuccessful attempt to falsify the theory. (I now speak in such cases of 'corroborating evidence').[11]

The following excerpts from a dialogue by Steve Williams[12] should illustrate the workings of hypothesis generation and testing, and also show that despite having found no 'obvious' falsification, one can be found at a later stage.[12] In fact the story shows that even apparently simple facts are much more complex. The story is about the discovery of vaccination against anthrax by Louis Pasteur. He 'proved' that anthrax vaccination prevents the outbreak of disease in a scientific experiment on only 25 sheep.

Paul. How could Pasteur know for sure that he'd found the right vaccine after trying it on only 25 sheep?

Laura. What do you mean?

Paul. Well, imagine if a big bin suddenly appeared on the school field. Because I'm brave I get to the bin first. I reach into the bin and pick out 25 things. They are all chocolate bars.

Daniel. Is this a dream you have every night or something?

Paul. Listen! The first 25 things are chocolate bars. How do I know the 26th thing won't be something else even a bomb? How did Pasteur know that 25 sheep would be enough to test his vaccine?

Gulnaz. But this is different. No sheep had ever survived anthrax before and there must have been thousands of deaths. The vaccinated sheep all survived.

Daniel. Yes, and every one of the other sheep who'd been injected with anthrax germs died. There's not much chance of that happening for no reason.

Kerrie. It fitted in with Pasteur's theory too. He could explain why it happened that way.

Louis Pasteur. You are right my friends, making discoveries in science is about having theories and then finding out whether things really happen that way. It's also about looking at something that happens and trying to think of a theory that explains it. It works both ways. But you ask interesting questions. Were 25 sheep enough to prove my theory? Make up your own minds. But imagine what it was like trying to persuade a farmer that I could stop his sheep getting anthrax by injecting them with anthrax. I was lucky to get any sheep to work on. But I was famous and that always helps.

The full dynamics of science are displayed. You start with an idea, you formulate a theory, you design an experiment to show – or more correctly verify – that your theory works, and you need charisma to defend your stance. Critics are easily silenced in the euphoria of the moment, sweeping aside the results of any other experiment that might contradict the new discovery.

Max Von Pettenkofer. Can I say something Louis?

Kerrie. Who are you?

Max Von Pettenkofer. Max Von Pettenkofer – a German scientist. I lived at the same time as Louis Pasteur.

Louis Pasteur. Max didn't believe that bacteria caused disease. He even drank a glass of water full of cholera bacteria to show his faith.

Max Von Pettenkofer. And I survived. Doesn't that prove something?

Critical discourse is needed as not to lose sight of the trees for the woods. The apparent verification of a cause and effect situation invariably occurs in a complex environment, and other factors may have an important influence on the outcomes observed.

Louis Pasteur. It proves you were very lucky. Haven't you kept in touch with the world since you died Max? Scientists agree that bacteria and other kinds of germs do cause diseases. Vaccines can help to stop diseases spreading.

Max Von Pettenkofer. I was wrong in some ways, but in some ways I was right. It depends what we mean by that word 'cause'. Why don't you tell them about the worms Louis and why one field was deadly to sheep but another was harmless.

Louis Pasteur. What are you getting at Max?

Max Von Pettenkofer. Let's hear the story. Then I'll explain.

Louis Pasteur. One day I was walking in a field of sheep. I noticed that the ground in one part of the field was a different colour to the rest. As I got closer, I noticed lots of worm casts – the soil worms push out as they tunnel along. I asked the farmer about this and he told me a few of his sheep had died of anthrax. He buried them in the field. I guessed that the worms had been feeding off the dead sheep. They brought the anthrax bacteria to the surface and the live sheep ate grass with the bacteria on it. But the anthrax could have been passed on in other ways. Sheep with cuts and scratches sometimes rubbed against other sheep with the disease.

Max Von Pettenkofer. So was anthrax caused by the bacteria or by the farmer burying the dead sheep in the field, or both? And did the farmer keep his sheep healthy enough? What do your young friends think?

Paul. A cause always comes just before the thing it causes. The bacteria getting into the sheep was the last thing to happen before they got ill so I think the bacteria is the cause.

Kerrie. But if the farmer hadn't buried the dead sheep with anthrax in the same field, the anthrax might not have spread. That set off the chain of events that got the anthrax into all the live sheep.

Gulnaz. Maybe there are more causes than one. These could both be causes in different ways.

Barry. Grass is the cause. It wouldn't have happened without grass.

Kerrie. Barry, what do you mean?

Barry. If there wasn't grass, the sheep wouldn't have eaten it – so no deadly bacteria.

Kerrie. They would just have died of starvation.

Gulnaz. Anyway, all sheep eat grass but not all sheep get anthrax. I think a cause must be something that doesn't happen all the time.

Louis Pasteur. We could go on saying it couldn't have happened except for this or that but the thing is it did. We needed a quick way to stop the disease spreading. Our methods worked. They've worked for many other diseases too.

Max Von Pettenkofer. You'll never get rid of all the germs in the world Louis. And even you have to admit that some vaccines don't work very well. There are other ways to stop germs spreading – by taking better care of ourselves and our animals. When people are able to keep clean and well-fed we see less disease; when they aren't we see more. We also know that healthy people and healthy animals can survive serious diseases – like I survived my drink of cholera. So in a way I was proved right.

Louis Pasteur. I agree Max, but we still need vaccines for times when things go wrong, and for people who are not strong and healthy.

Max Von Pettenkofer. Maybe you are right. But at least our young friends have plenty to think and ask questions about.

Louis Pasteur. That's one thing we all have in common. We always liked to ask questions and asking good questions is the way to make discoveries. That will never change.

Scientific research can ever only lead to a better approximation of the truth.

HOW SCIENCE WORKS

Don Mikulecky, a physiologist at the Medical College of Virginia Commonwealth University, analysed the mental mechanism underpinning science. Science builds *formal models* that help us to understand the *real world* around us. The natural system is encoded into an experimental formal system; the causalities in the natural system are simulated by manipulations and implications within the formal system, and the resulting changes in the formal system are then decoded back to the natural system. If we find that the two systems hang together we consider our 'scientific' model to be a valid explanation of the real world (*see* Figure 7.1).[13]

THE PARADIGM OF SCIENCE

The truth of a theory is in your mind, not in your eyes.

Albert Einstein[15]

What most experimenters take for granted before they begin their experiments is infinitely more interesting than any results to which their experiments lead.

Norbert Wiener

The notion of the scientific paradigm was introduced by Thomas Kuhn (1922–1996) to describe the observation that at any time in history, science followed a particular theoretical framework. This framework draws together the mental mindset, the questions and the methods of scientists in a particular field. In an accepted framework, researchers can safely focus all their attention on small questions, solving puzzles, without the need to question the underlying assumptions of their field of study. Within a given paradigm researchers are working to verify their theories, acting contrary to Popper's notion of falsification as the real basis of scientific work.

Hence, if a result does not completely fit the assumptions of the framework, researchers tend to make allowances to accommodate these findings rather than

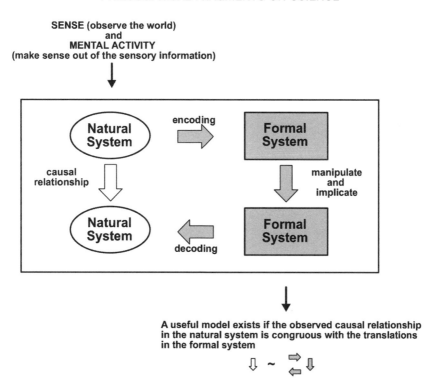

SENSE (observe the world)
and
MENTAL ACTIVITY
(make sense out of the sensory information)

Figure 7.1   How science works (adapted from Mikulecky[13] and Ferreira[14]).

challenging their framework as such. Only if findings accumulate or are so significantly in disagreement with the paradigm of the time, a crisis occurs, destabilising and traumatising the field and its workers.

Ultimately and under great psychological distress, a new paradigm emerges, built on new assumptions and new theories, until the entire field has stabilised with a new identity, e.g. the shift from classical mechanics to relativity theory, and further to quantum mechanics. When established, researchers revert back to the same approach to their work as they have done under the previous paradigm.[16]

The whole paradigm of reductionist science has been challenged by physicists themselves; Bob Laughlin started his 1998 Nobel Prize Lecture highlighting his conclusion with this example:

> One of my favourite times in the academic year occurs in early spring when I give my class of extremely bright graduate students, who have mastered quantum mechanics but are otherwise unsuspecting and innocent, a take-home exam in which they are asked to deduce superfluidity from first principles. There is no doubt a very special place in hell being reserved for me at this very moment for this mean trick, for the task is impossible. Superfluidity, like the fractional Hall effect, is an emergent phenomenon – a low-energy collective effect of huge numbers of particles that cannot be deduced from the microscopic equations of motion in a rigorous way, and that disappears completely when

the system is taken apart. There are prototypes for superfluids, of course, and students who memorize them have taken the first step down the long road to understanding the phenomenon, but these are all approximate and in the end not deductive at all, but fits to experiment. The students feel betrayed and hurt by this experience because they have been trained to think in reductionist terms and thus to believe that everything that is not amenable to such thinking is unimportant. But nature is much more heartless than I am, and those students who stay in physics long enough to seriously confront the experimental record eventually come to understand that the reductionist idea is wrong a great deal of the time, and perhaps always . . . The world is full of things for which one's understanding, i.e. one's ability to predict what will happen in an experiment, is degraded by taking the system apart, including most delightfully the standard model of elementary particles itself. I myself have come to suspect that all the important outstanding problems in physics are emergent in nature, including in particular quantum gravity.[17]

THE PARADIGM OF MEDICAL SCIENCE

At most medical schools the undergraduate curriculum is divided into 'basic sciences' and 'clinical sciences'. In all cases it is taken for granted that medicine is a scientific pursuit.

Science has been divided into basic and applied forms. The definition of basic, Feinstein observed, is based more on the minuteness of the matter than the magnitude of the problem, and that science has often been defined by its goal rather than its method.[18] Based on this perception he concluded that those amongst us who study man, rather than his cells, can never be regarded as basic scientists.

For the clinical context Reiser concluded:

> [for] too many doctors, the laboratory 'seemed pervaded by a purer light' than the hospital ward, and the laboratory analyst was pictured as superior to the clinician – 'the incarnation of all that is scientific in medicine and whose word cannot be questioned.'[19]

Science and technology have become closely related in the 20th century. Science is concerned with knowledge, technology with power. The distinction between science and technology is often not clear any more. Whereas science asks 'Is it true?', technology asks 'Does it work?'. McWhinney raises concerns about the consequences of the latter question. He asks another question:

> 'Work for what?' There is always, therefore, potential conflict between technological and other human values.[20]

This latter point is clearly consistent with Laughlin's conclusion that the parts alone are not sufficient to understanding a discipline – there are the scientific facts of medicine, but there are also the human facts of medicine, and the facts defined by the personal understanding of the patient about his illness. The knowledge of the field of medicine is broader than the knowledge about the biological parts of the human body.

KNOWLEDGE

There are all kinds of sources of our knowledge but none has authority.

Karl Popper[11]

We know more than we can tell.

Michael Polanyi[21]

Where is the life we have lost in living? Where is the wisdom we have lost in
knowledge? Where is the knowledge we have lost in information?

TS Eliot[22]

What is knowledge? Knowledge is information we are aware of and can be classified
as *knowing what* – naming facts and relationships – and *knowing how* – explaining
procedures.

Knowledge has also been classified as explicit knowledge, which can be codified
and can be easily communicated, and tacit knowledge, which cannot be codified and
therefore cannot be easily passed on to others.

It is perhaps pragmatic to use Michael Polanyi's (1891–1976) explanations. He used
the term tacit knowledge to describe the domain of personal knowing.[21] Tacit knowing
has been further divided into a technical dimension – also described as know-how
and arising from a wealth of experience, though being hard to explain or transfer, and
a cognitive dimension consisting of beliefs, perceptions, ideals, values, emotions and
mental models. It is this tacit knowledge that largely shapes the way we perceive the
world around us. In relation to medical sciences Polanyi stated that:

> ... personal knowledge in science is not made but discovered, and as such it claims
> to establish contact with reality beyond the clues on which it relies. It commits us,
> passionately and far beyond our comprehension, to a vision of reality. Of this responsibility
> we cannot divest ourselves by setting up objective criteria of verifiability – or falsifiability,
> or testability, or what you will. For we live in it as in the garment of our own skin.[21]

For Polanyi, tacit and explicit are different but inseparable aspects of knowledge.[23] Both
can be learnt though the learning modes will be different. Tacit knowledge is largely
transferred in an experiential way in apprenticeship situations.[23,24]

KNOWLEDGE MANAGEMENT AND KNOWLEDGE TRANSFER

Philosophically knowledge was seen as a *thing* in the Kantian tradition and as such *was
waiting there to be discovered*. However this view has significant deficiencies that became
ever more apparent through the impact of the science of complex adaptive systems in
the late 1990s. In a complex adaptive systems framework, knowledge in addition to
being a *thing* simultaneously also is a *flow*, as the focus of knowledge generation shifts
primarily to *context* and *narrative*, rather than content alone.[25] Snowden illustrates how
these changes effect knowledge management [in organisations] through these three
heuristics:

1   *knowledge can only be volunteered; it cannot be conscripted* for the very simple reason that I can never truly know if someone is using his or her knowledge. I can know they have complied with a process or a quality standard. But, we have trained managers to manage conscripts not volunteers

2   *we can always know more than we can tell, and we will always tell more than we can write down.* The nature of knowledge is such that we always know, or are capable of knowing more than we have the physical time or the conceptual ability to say. I can speak in five minutes what it will otherwise take me two weeks to get round to spend a couple of hours writing it down. The process of writing something down is reflective knowledge; it involves both adding and taking away from the actual experience or original thought. Reflective knowledge has high value, but is time consuming and involves loss of control over its subsequent use

3   *we only know what we know when we need to know it,* human knowledge is deeply contextual, it is triggered by circumstance. In understanding what people know we have to recreate the context of their knowing if we were to ask a meaningful question or enable knowledge use. To ask someone what he or she knows is to ask a meaningless question in a meaningless context, but such approaches are at the heart of mainstream consultancy method.[25]

GAINING KNOWLEDGE THROUGH SENSE MAKING

Kurtz and Snowden described knowledge generation and knowledge management as a sense-making process.[26] They used the Welsh word *cynefin* (pronounced kun-ev'in), which has no direct English translation, to describe both – the state as well as the process – of knowledge generation and sense making. They describe the meaning of *Cynefin* as follows:

> It is more properly understood as the place of our multiple affiliations, the sense that we all, individually and collectively, have many roots, cultural, religious, geographic, tribal, and so forth. We can never be fully aware of the nature of those affiliations, but they profoundly influence what we are. The name seeks to remind us that all human interactions are strongly influenced and frequently determined by the patterns of our multiple experiences, both through the direct influence of personal experience and through collective experience expressed as stories.[26]

The Cynefin model of knowledge and sense making synthesises all of the meanings of knowledge and provides a framework to understanding knowledge as a personal construct, consisting of *things and flows* – describing facts and describing the struggle to reaching personal knowing.

Kurtz and Snowden used the Cynefin model to describe the different knowledge domains – the known, the knowable, the complex or emerging, and the chaotic or random – and their relationships to human thinking and organisational management.

Figure 7.2 translates 'medicine' into this framework. It becomes apparent that we always operate in all domains some of the time, or move to and from one domain to another depending on our current context.

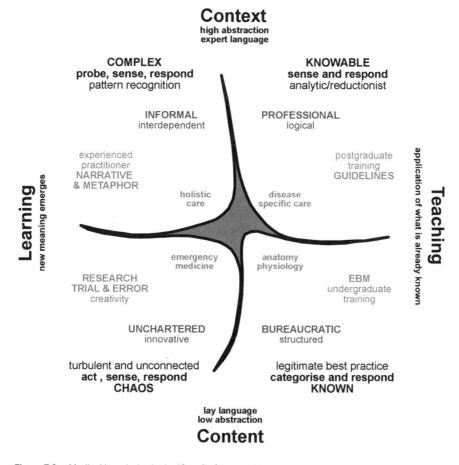

Figure 7.2   Medical knowledge in the 'Cynefin framework'.

The figure has tried to translate our knowledge, our professional development, our mode of action, our tools and our organisational affiliations into the Cynefin model. It should be firstly noted that each of the four domains uses different thinking strategies to problem solving, secondly that the domains are value-free, neither is intrinsically better than any other, and thirdly all domains are interdependent.

Figure 7.3 illustrates the *flow* dimension of the process of knowledge generation; knowledge is produced through a perpetual process that at times leads to an end-product, a temporarily static 'known fact' within a given paradigm. As more knowledge is generated, current facts become superseded by new ones.

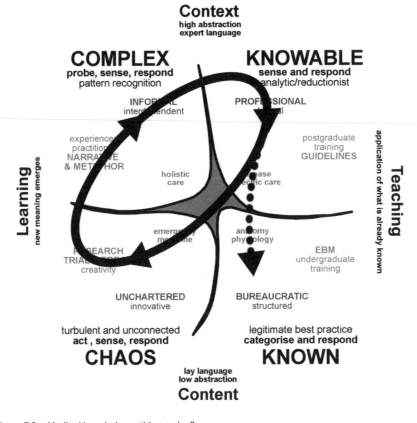

Figure 7.3 Medical knowledge: a thing and a flow.

SUMMARY POINTS

- The Cartesian concept of mind and body promoted the adoption of the body-machine metaphor.
- The adoption of the notion that understanding the parts imparts knowledge about the whole is reflected in deductive reasoning and has become the rationale for reductionist thinking.
- Observation is always selective since it always requires a chosen object.
- Failure to falsify a hypothesis makes it a strong hypothesis.
- Scientific results are approximations of the truth, not the truth itself.
- A paradigm is an accepted mental framework under which scientists conduct their experiments.
- The reductionist paradigm of science is no longer supported by the results of scientific work.
- Knowledge has explicit and tacit components.
- Knowledge is both a thing and a flow, and knowledge generation a sense-making process.

CHAPTER 8

Systems thinking

Always think of the Universe as one living organism, with a single substance, and a single soul; and observe how all things are submitted to the single perceptivity of this one whole; all are moved by its single impulse, and all play their part in the causation of every event that happens. Remark the intricacy of the skein, and the complexity of the web.

Marcus Aurelius, the Roman Emperor and Stoic philosopher [27]

For every problem there is one solution which is simple, neat and wrong.

HL Mencken, satirist

The Newtonian paradigm, like all other past, present and future paradigms, is only an approximation of reality, and thus transient and limited. As we learn about the reality around us we discover more hidden patterns of nature, and we experience the emergences of new understandings and changing worldviews.[28]

The Newtonian paradigm propelled advances in the physical sciences leading to the development of technologies, and the rapid economic advances associated with the industrial revolution. At the same time it suppressed critical thought and hindered the development of the life sciences.[8,28]

Newton's views were already challenged during his life, e.g. by the French philosopher Denis Diderot (1713–1784) who wrote:

Look at this egg: with it you can overthrow all the schools of theology and all the churches in the world. What is this egg? An insensitive mass before the germ is put into it . . . How does this mass evolve into a new organization, into sensitivity, into life? Through heat. What will generate heat in it? Motion. What will the successive effects of motion be? Instead of answering me, sit down and let us follow out these effects with our eyes from one moment to the next. First there is a speck which moves about, a thread growing and taking colour, flesh being formed, a beak, wing-tips, eyes, feet coming into view, a yellowish substance which unwinds and turns into intestines – and you have a living creature . . . Now the wall is breached and the bird emerges, walks, flies, feels pain, runs away, comes back again, complains, suffers, loves, desires, enjoys, it experiences all your affections and does all the things you do. And will you maintain with Descartes that it is an imitating machine pure and simple? Why, even little children will laugh at you, and philosophers will answer that if it is a machine you are one too! If, however, you admit that the only difference between you and an animal is one of organization, you will be showing sense and reason and be acting in good faith; but then it will be concluded, contrary to what you had said, that from an inert substance arranged in a certain way and impregnated by another inert substance, subjected to heat and motion, you will get sensitivity, life, memory, consciousness, passions, thought . . . Just listen to your own arguments and you will feel how pitiful they are. You will come to feel that by refusing to entertain a simple hypothesis that explains everything – sensitivity as a property common to all matter or as a result of the organization of matter – you are flying in the face of common sense and plunging into a chasm of mysteries, contradictions and absurdities. (cited in reference 28)

TABLE 8.1 The differences between the analytic and systemic worldview (adapted from J de Rosnay. *Analytic vs. Systemic Approaches*[30])

ANALYTIC/REDUCTIONIST APPROACH	SYSTEMIC/HOLISTIC APPROACH
Aim	
Explain the whole through the properties of its parts, e.g. the human body can be understood through its organs and cells	Explain the whole through the arrangement and relationships of its parts, e.g. societies can be understood through the relationships of their individuals
Approach	
• Isolates, then concentrates on the elements	• Unifies and concentrates on the interaction between elements
• Studies the nature of interaction	• Studies the effects of interactions
• Emphasises the precision of details	• Emphasises global perception
• Modifies one variable at a time	• Modifies groups of variables simultaneously
• Remains independent of duration of time; the phenomena considered are reversible	• Integrates duration of time and irreversibility
• Validates facts by means of experimental proof within the body of a theory	• Validates facts through comparison of the behaviour of the model with reality
• Has an efficient approach when interactions are linear and weak	• Has an efficient approach when interactions are non-linear and strong
• Leads to discipline-oriented (juxtadisciplinary) education	• Leads to multidisciplinary education
• Leads to action programmed in detail	• Leads to action through objectives
• Possesses knowledge of details, poorly defined goals	• Possesses knowledge of goals, fuzzy details

The Cartesian worldview has been the subconscious template for seeing all things around us in a mechanistic or clockwork fashion. However there now is a growing insight that understanding the whole through its parts is not sustainable, which has led to the proposition that the whole is better understood through the arrangement and the relationships of the parts, the foundation of systems and complexity thinking.[8] Table 8.1 compares the perspectives of the two approaches.[28,29]

Systems theory goes back to the 1940s and 1950s and emerged from the interdisciplinary thinking of the American mathematician Norbert Wiener (1894–1964), the Austrian biologist Ludwig von Bertalanffy (1901–1972), the British psychiatrist Ross Ashby (1903–1972) and the Austrian physicist and philosopher Heinz von Foerster (1911–2002). Other important thinkers in the field include Ilya Prigogine (1917–2003) who introduced the concept of dissipative structures, and Humberto Maturana (born 1928) and Francisco Varela (1946–2001) who introduced the concept of autopoiesis.

General systems theory, proposed in the 1940s by van Bertalanffy states that:

- real systems are open to, and interact with their environments
- they can acquire qualitatively new properties through emergence, resulting in continual evolution
- systems focus on the arrangement of and relations between the parts which connect them into a whole.

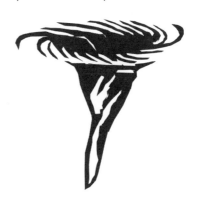

Prigogine proposed that living systems are dissipative structures. The emphasis of a dissipative structure is on the openness of the structure to the flow of energy or matter, i.e. despite the constant changes the structure remains stable, and it does so autonomously through self-organisation. A good everyday example of a dissipative structure is a vortex; despite all the activity occurring in it, it remains stable, and even when you disturb it, still will return to its original structure.

COMPLEX ADAPTIVE SYSTEMS

To understand complex adaptive systems one should think about them as having three conceptual dimensions – pattern, structure and process.[31] The pattern describes the configuration of relationships that determine the system's essential characteristics (one may think of it like the architectural drawing of a building); the structure of the system is made up of its physical components (the bricks, roof tiles, power points, etc.), and the process describes the activities within the system (people moving around and engaging themselves within the building, e.g. holding conversations, cooking and eating, changing the furniture and so on), all of which is *at the same time* determined and constrained by the pattern or design of and the structure or physical state (of the building).

Box 8.1 describes some of the important characteristics of a complex adaptive system, and Figure 8.1 summaries the characteristics and behaviours of complex systems graphically.

BOX 8.1 Characteristics of complex adaptive systems (adapted from C Joslyn *The Nature of Cybernetic Systems*[32])

- *Complexity*: heterogeneous interacting components, e.g. organisms, societies, ecologies
- *Mutuality*: interactions occur in parallel, co-operatively and in real time, creating simultaneous interactions
- *Complementarity*: interactions lead to subsystems that interact in multiple processes
- *Evolvability*: complex adaptive systems tend to evolve and grow opportunistically
- Constructivity: as a complex adaptive system increases in size and complexity, it becomes historically bound to previous states while simultaneously developing new traits
- *Reflexivity*: complex adaptive systems are rich in internal and external feedback loops, that ultimately allow self-reference, self-modelling, self-production and self-reproduction

---

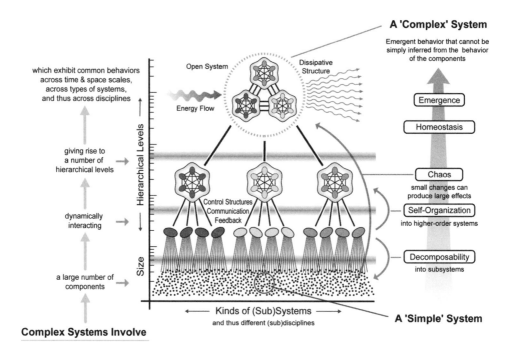

Figure 8.1 Characteristics and behaviours of complex adaptive systems. Complex adaptive systems, through self-organisation, are structured in a hierarchical fashion; they interact across their subsystem boundaries, and over time, through co-evolution, emerge towards new states (figure kindly provided by Marshal Clemens from idiagram - www.idiagram.com).

The following sections will reiterate the concepts of complex adaptive systems in clinical care. At this point some examples should illustrate the applicability of the concepts in health and disease:

- The human body is composed of multiple interacting and self-regulating physiological systems including biochemical and neuroendocrine feedback loops.
- The behaviour of any individual is determined partly by an internal set of rules based on past experience and partly by unique and adaptive responses to new stimuli from the environment.
- The web of relationships in which individuals exist contains many varied and powerful determinants of their beliefs, expectations and behaviour.
- Individuals and their immediate social relationships are further embedded within wider social, political and cultural systems which can influence outcomes in entirely novel and unpredictable ways.
- All these interacting systems are dynamic and fluid.
- A small change in one part of this web of interacting systems may lead to a much larger change in another part through amplification effects.[33]

SUMMARY POINTS

- General systems theory states that adaptive systems are open to, and interact with their environment, that they can acquire qualitatively new properties through emergence, resulting in continual evolution, and that the system focus is on the arrangement of and relations between the parts which connect them into a whole.
- Living systems are dissipative structures, i.e. the structure remains stable despite the constant changes within. This stability occurs autonomously through self-organisation.
- Complex adaptive system have three conceptual dimensions – pattern, structure and process.

CHAPTER 9

Emerging patterns

> Both medicine and philosophy as dialogue begin with an inter-human event. This inter-human event is . . . the locus of meaning . . . Both philosophy and medicine share a common function as a dialectic of human beings . . . In this way, MEANING, including historical meaning, is imminent in the inter-human event. This is the locus of philosophy. Similarly medicine begins with a dialectic of human beings, a dialogue about sickness and health. From this the inter-human event both disciplines develop.
>
> *Pellegrino and Thomasma*[1]

This section has identified three patterns that are important in the understanding of medicine and primary care. Much of what we see as *common knowledge* is engrained in society's subconscious understanding of their lifeworld. Part of that *common knowledge* is the construction of health and illness around the notion of health being a balanced state, and illness being the loss of that balance. The role of the doctor is to make sense out of the experience of loss, and to help restore the balance of health.

A second strand engrained in our *common knowledge* is the acceptance of the mind–body split and the mechanistic/clockwork understanding of the workings of the body and nature at large. Implicit in this model is the notion that every phenomenon can be understood by breaking it down into its constituent parts, and that understanding the parts will allow an understanding of the whole. This reductionist paradigm has many deficiencies and is slowly crumbling to be replaced by a scientific model that views phenomena in the context of a greater whole and that acknowledges that the world is not predictable – the complex adaptive systems model.

And lastly we are gaining an understanding that knowledge is a personal construct that provides us with meaning – meanings change over time, and knowledge hence has to be viewed simultaneously as being *fixed facts* and *constant flow*. Knowledge itself is a complex adaptive system.

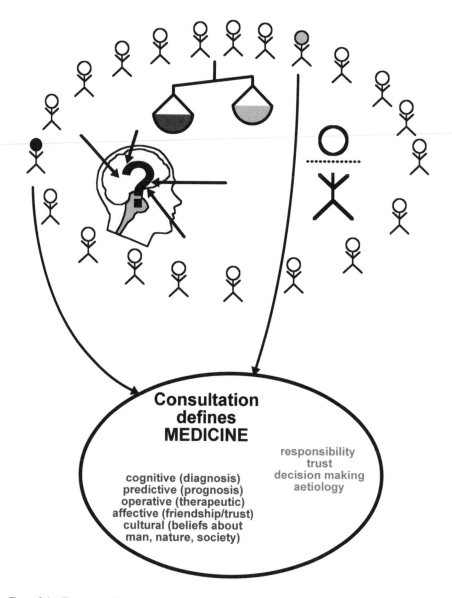

Figure 9.1 The pattern of understanding medicine. Inherent in society's sub/consciousness are three notions: illness is a loss of balance; the mind–body split drives medical sciences; and knowing is a complex personal phenomenon. The historical primacy of the consultation remains the defining characteristic of medicine as a discipline.

Figure 9.1 illustrates how these understandings define and affect the practice of medicine. In particular they fit with the historical understanding of the primacy of the consultation. And as Pellegrino and Thomasma have shown, the defining characteristic of the discipline of medicine is the interaction of doctor and patient in the clinical encounter.

Medicine does, in fact, derive much of its method, logic, and theory from the physical and biological sciences, so it is to a certain extent a branch of those sciences. But medicine is also a praxis in the Aristotelian sense – knowledge applied for human ends and purposes. In this sense, medicine can be classed among the technologies. But medicine also sets out to modify the behavior of individuals and societies, and thus has roots in the behavioral sciences. Finally, medicine operates through a personal, and therefore an ethical, relationship intended to 'help' the person to 'better' health. It is a value-laden activity, with roots in ethics and the humanities.[1]

Medicine, even as science, must encompass the special complexities of man as subject interacting with man as object of science. Physiology, unlike the clinical science of medicine, studies physical processes while ignoring the lived reality of the experimental subject – his or her self-perceived history, uniqueness, and individuality. Thus even when it functions as clinical science, medicine must correlate the explanatory modes of the physical sciences with those of the social and behavioral.[1]

FURTHER READING

Capra F. *The Web of Life*. London: Harper Collins Publishers, 1996.

Heylighen F, Cilliers P and Gershenson C. *Complexity and Philosophy*. http://uk.arxiv.org/pdf/cs.CC/0604072 (accessed 30 June 2006).

Kleinman A. *Patients and Healers in the Context of Cultures*. Los Angeles: University of California Press, 1980.

Kurtz C and Snowden D. The new dynamics of strategy: sense-making in a complex and complicated world. *IBM Systems Journal*. 2003; **42**: 462–83.

Pellegrino E and Thomasma D. *A Philosophical Basis of Medical Practice. Towards a philosophy and ethic of the healing professions*. New York, Oxford: Oxford University Press, 1981.

Popper K. *Conjectures and Refutations: the growth of scientific knowledge*. London: Routledge and Kegan Paul, 1972.

REFERENCES

1 Pellegrino E and Thomasma D. *A Philosophical Basis of Medical Practice. Towards a philosophy and ethic of the healing professions*. New York, Oxford: Oxford University Press, 1981.

2 Moes M. Plato's conception of the relationship between moral philosophy and medicine. *Perspectives in Biology and Medicine*. 2001; **44**: 353–67.

3 Stoyan-Rosenzweig N. *Balancing the Humors: healing traditions and medical practice in world medicine*. http://medinfo.ufl.edu/other/histmed/stoyan2/ (accessed 30 June 2006).

4 Kleinman A. Culture and illness: a question of models [editorial]. *Culture, Medicine and Psychiatry*. 1977; **1**: 229–31.

5 Duncan W. Caring or curing: conflicts of choice. *Journal of the Royal Society of Medicine*. 1985; **78**: 526–35.

6 Lewis C. *Exploring the biological meaning of disease and health*. www.chester.ac.uk/~sjlewis/DM/Vienna.htm (accessed 30 June 2006).

7 Kleinman A. *Patients and Healers in the Context of Cultures*. Los Angeles: University of California Press, 1980.

8 Heylighen F, Cilliers P and Gershenson C. *Complexity and Philosophy*. http://uk.arxiv.org/pdf/cs.CC/0604072 (accessed 30 June 2006).

9 Saul JR. *The Unconscious Civilization*. Ringwood, Australia: Penguin Books, 1997.

10 Brecht B. *The Life of Galileo*. London: Eyre Methuen, 1980.

11 Popper K. *Conjectures and Refutations: the growth of scientific knowledge*. London: Routledge and Kegan Paul, 1972.

12 Williams S. *The Science of Louis Pasteur*. www.dialogueworks.co.uk/dw/wr/past1.html (accessed 30 June 2006).

13 Mikulecky D. *If the Whole World is Complex – Why Bother?* www.people.vcu.edu/~mikuleck/alskuniv.htm (accessed 30 June 2006).

14 Ferreira P. *Tracing Complexity Theory*. star.tau.ac.il/~eshel/Bio_complexity/ 7.Complexity/Complexity%20Theory.ppt (accessed 30 June 2005).

15 Eves H. *Mathematical Circles Squared*. Boston: Prindle, Weber and Schmidt, 1972.

16 Kuhn T. *The Structure of Scientific Revolutions*. Chicago: University of Chicago Press, 1970.

17 Laughlin R. *Fractional Quantization*. Nobel Lecture, 1998. http://nobelprize.org/physics/laureates/1998/laughlin-lecture.html (accessed 30 June 2006).

18 Feinstein A. *Clinical Judgement*. New York: The Williams & Wilkins Company, 1967.

19 Reiser S. *The Shortcomings of Technology*. Cambridge: Cambridge University Press, 1982.

20 McWhinney I. Medical knowledge and the rise of technology. *Journal of Medicine and Philosophy*. 1978; **3**: 293–304.

21 Polanyi M. *Tacit Dimension*. New York: Anchor Books, 1967.

22 Eliot TS. The Rock. In: TS Eliot. *Complete Poems and Plays: 1909–1950*. London: Harcourt, 1952. p. 48.

23 Polanyi M. *Personal Knowledge. Towards a post-critical philosophy*. London: Routledge, 1958.

24 Wyatt J. Management of explicit and tacit knowledge. *Journal of the Royal Society of Medicine*. 2001; **94**: 6–9.

25 Snowden D. Complex acts of knowing: paradox and descriptive self-awareness. *Journal of Knowledge Management*. 2002; **6**(2): 100–11.

26 Kurtz C and Snowden D. The new dynamics of strategy: sense-making in a complex and complicated world. *IBM Systems Journal*. 2003; **42**: 462–83.

27 Marcus Aurelius. *Meditations. Book 5*. London: Penguin, 1964.

28 Kurakin A. *Watchmaker versus Self-Organization. Part I. Critique of the Newtonian worldview*. www.alexeikurakin.org/text/ak112103.pdf (accessed 30 June 2006).

29 Mikulecky D. Definition of Complexity. www.people.vcu.edu/~mikuleck/ON%20COMPLEXITY. (accessed 30 June 2006).

30 de Rosnay J. *Analytic vs. Systemic Approaches*. In: F Heylighen, C Joslyn and V Turchin (eds): *Principia Cybernetica Web*. Brussels, Principia Cybernetica. http://pespmc1.vub.ac.be/ANALSYST.html (accessed 30 June 2006).

31 Capra F. *The Web of Life*. London: HarperCollins Publishers, 1996.

32 Joslyn C. *The Nature of Cybernetic Systems*. In: F Heylighen, C Joslyn and V Turchin (eds): *Principia Cybernetica Web*. Brussels, Principia Cybernetica. http://pespmc1.vub.ac.be\CYBSNAT.html (accessed 30 June 2006).

33 Wilson T and Holt T. Complexity and clinical care. *British Medical Journal*. 2001; **323**: 685–8.

History   Philosophy   The Practice of Medicine   Social   Primary Care

Social Construct of Health
Public Health Infrastructure

Shaman/Medicine Man
Hippocrates of Cos
Care for the Whole Patient

Broad Education
Apprenticeship Model
of Learning

Knowledge of Disease
School of Cnidus

Husserl

Pellegrino

Cynefin Knowledge Model

Cartesian ←——→ Complexity
Dualism

Popper

Personal Relationship
Phronesis
Continuity of Care
Care Co-ordination
Quality of Life

SOMATIC
SOCIAL — PSYCHOLOGICAL
SEMIOTIC

Science & Technology

Social
Capital

Income
Inequality

Employment

Access

Common Goal
Integrated BUT
Diverse Solutions

Personal
Health Gain

SECTION THREE

The practice of medicine: healing

In particular I believe that cure is rare while the need for care is widespread, and that the pursuit of cure at all costs may restrict the supply of care, but the bias has at least been declared.

Archie Cochrane[61]

Medical care – who determines what it is, and how is it negotiated between patients and doctors? It is an important question to reflect upon – particularly in light of the philosophical foundations of medicine. Is there a unifying model of health and health care that overcomes the Cartesian reductionism of the past centuries?

Healing is the ultimate goal of medicine. Illness, rather than disease, brings the patient to the doctor. Many illnesses are not associated with a definable disease, and the classical model of *curing a disease* does not apply to *healing of the illness*. Healing is the process of coming to terms with one's illness, making sense of that experience in light of one's life circumstances. The relationship between the doctor and the patient creates the therapeutic environment for healing.

The first chapter in this section describes the epidemiology of illness and disease in the community. Illness is common, disease is rare. However the fear of illness and disease has increased markedly over the past 40 years despite the fact that we never experienced better health ever.

The second chapter explores the related but distinctive notions of disease, illness and health. Disease is social in nature, whereas illness and disease is of a personal nature. A dynamic balance model of health is proposed that integrates the somatic, mental, social and sense-making (semiotic) aspects of the health and illness experience, and offers a means to overcome the prevailing Cartesian dualism in health care.

Medicine needs to re-emphasise the need to care. The third chapter argues that medicine must adapt its limited knowledge in the context of a unique understanding of our patients' needs. Care is based on a personal relationship between the doctor and his patient. This relationship is informed by the diverse knowledge arising from psychoneuroimmunology, technology and evidence-based medicine, all of which affect the process and the outcome of care.

The final chapter examines general practice/family medicine in more detail. The discipline is defined in relationship terms and by its commitment to the person in his community. The personal relationship between doctor and patient enhances the consultation through patient centredness, trust, knowledge about each other and, ultimately, wise clinical decisions. The ongoing relationship provides much-needed stability in a rapidly changing healthcare system, equally benefiting patients and the system.

CHAPTER 10

The epidemiology of illness and disease

> Every scientific truth goes through three states: first, people say it conflicts with the Bible; next, they say it has been discovered before. Lastly, they say they always believed it.
>
> *Louis Agassiz (1807–1873)*

How healthy are the people in our community? Looking at all the media hype about the threats caused by old and emerging diseases we all must be on guard all the time.

How true are these threats really? How much are we influenced by the constant bombardment of threat in our environment? Are we as doctors fuelling the fear of disease, and the vulnerability to succumb to them? Shouldn't the fact that we survived the evolutionary pressures in pretty good shape be reassuring?

There are two ways of assessing the health state of a community, one by looking at mortality statistics, the other by asking people to report on their health and their responses to experiencing illness.

Mortality statistics have one big irony; we all are going to be one at some stage. The accuracy of mortality statistics is limited by the fact that they are largely compiled on the basis of clinical rather than post-mortem assessments. Mortality data nevertheless are helpful for the planning of health service priorities (*see* Table 10.1), but they do not tell us anything about the impact of the underlying disease(s) on life. In particular, mortality statistics do not help us in understanding and dealing with a particular patient's illness experience in the consultation.

TABLE 10.1 Leading causes of death: Australia and Fiji[1,2]

AUSTRALIA[a]	FIJI[b]
Malignancies	Diseases of the circulatory system
Ischaemic heart disease	Ill-defined conditions
Cerebrovascular disease	Hypertensive disease
Influenza and pneumonia	Ischaemic heart disease
Heart failure	Acute myocardial infarction
Hypertensive disease	Diabetes mellitus
Renal failure	Cerebrovascular disease
Chronic lower respiratory diseases	Nephritis, nephrotic syndrome
Diabetes mellitus	Malignancies
Organic, including symptomatic, mental disorders	Pneumonia

a Causes of Death 2003: Australian Bureau of Statistics[1]
b Causes of Death 2000: Fiji Islands Bureau of Statistics[2]

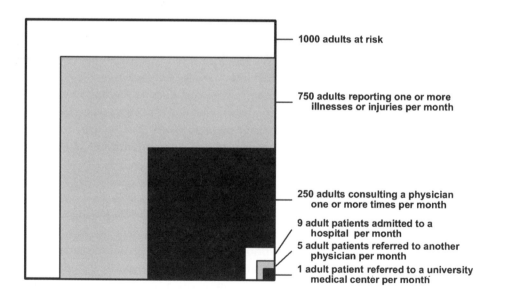

1000 adults at risk

750 adults reporting one or more illnesses or injuries per month

250 adults consulting a physician one or more times per month

9 adult patients admitted to a hospital per month

5 adult patients referred to another physician per month

1 adult patient referred to a university medical center per month

Figure 10.1 Monthly prevalence estimates of illness in the community and the roles of physicians, hospitals, and university medical centres in the provision of medical care. (Reproduced from White K, Williams F and Greenberg B. The ecology of medical care. *New England Journal of Medicine.* 1961; **265**: 885–92,[3] with permission from the Massachusetts Medical Society.)

White and colleagues explored the health and illness experience of the community and described a rather bright picture – most members of a community perceive themselves to be healthy and able to cope by themselves with most minor illness symptoms. Only a small percentage of those seeking medical care are subsequently diagnosed with a disease and/or require specialised medical services (*see* Figure 10.1).[3]

Community health and illness has changed little between 1961 and 2001. Larry Green and colleagues reviewed current data, and found that many more patients experience some illness symptoms and that about 30% more people seek care, mostly from complementary and alternative medical care providers.[4] These changes may well reflect the impact of the media hype alluded to above. There also has been a shift towards ambulatory/community care reflecting to some extent the needs of an aging population, and to another our greater ability to provide care based on technological advances. However, the number of patients requiring hospital care remains unchanged (*see* Figure 10.2).

It is rather remarkable how stable the epidemiology of disease has been over these four decades. It is equally remarkable to see that at a time when the population at large has never been healthier, the population also appears to be more afraid than ever of illness and death.[5] Figure 10.3 illustrates an analysis of the community's health-seeking behaviour – two questions of great importance arise: 'How did the community's perception of being ill change?' and 'How do individuals decide when and whom to consult when perceiving the need for medical care?'.

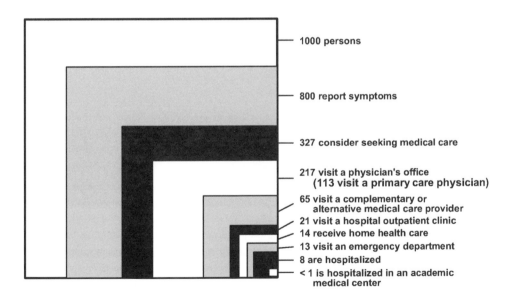

Figure 10.2 Re-analysis of the monthly prevalence of illness in the community and the roles of various sources of health care. (Reproduced form Green L, Fryer G, Yawn B, Lanier D and Dovey S. The ecology of medical care revisited. *New England Journal of Medicine.* 2001; **344**: 2021–5,[4] with permission from the Massachusetts Medical Society.)

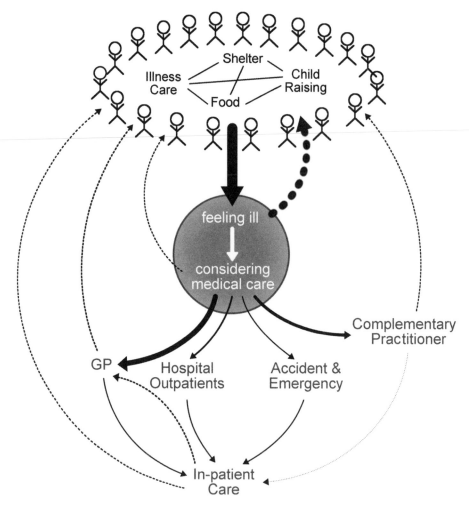

Figure 10.3 Care-seeking in the community: experiencing illness is common, seeking care is much less common.

SUMMARY POINTS

- Over the past 45 years the illness experience within Western communities has increased significantly; however, the incidence of serious disease has remained stable.
- People never lived a longer and more disability-free life ever; however, they appear to be more fearful of illness and death.

CHAPTER 11

Disease, illness and health

It is more important to know what patient has a disease, than what disease the patient has.

Sir William Osler

Each man has his particular way of being in good health.

Emanuel Kant

The focus of medicine has shifted beyond the question of an art or a science. No one doubts that sciences have improved our understanding of disease; however, patients do not experience diseases, they only experience the consequences of these.[6] Every patient is unique, and no two patients share the same illness narrative even if they have the same disease label.

Illness describes a subjective experience; it is the patient's account about his state of self.[7] Disease, in contrast, is the objective state of physical alteration, defined by abnormal measurements or pathological changes. It is time to rediscover this important distinction.

DISEASE

DISEASE: A SOCIAL CONSTRUCT

Disease is a social construct, constantly re-defined and re-interpreted.

Disease is at once a biological event, a generation-specific repertoire of verbal constructs reflecting medicine's intellectual and institutional history, an aspect of and potential legitimation for public policy, a potentially defining element of social role, a sanction for cultural norms, and a structuring element in doctor/patient interactions.[6]

Strictly speaking a disease only exists after we have agreed it does. A pathophysiological abnormality (e.g. bronchial hyper-reactivity) is not a disease as such, and not in everyone with the abnormality, it only is a disease after we have decided to call it asthma in those who show typical clinical features.[8]

Disease, as expressed in the *diagnosis*, is the central focus of modern medicine. Most of our education and most of our engagement with the patient is focused on establishing the diagnosis, i.e. defining the disease, before initiating specific therapeutic interventions.

Disease is also the basis for resource allocation and health service planning,[9] and the 'more popular' the status of a disease, e.g. HIV/AIDS, breast cancer or avian influenza, the more successful it will be in receiving scarce research funds.

DISEASE: A DIAGNOSIS

What do we mean by the term diagnosis? The Greek *dia* means by and *gnosis* means cognition/knowledge; however the term diagnosis had only been used sporadically until the 18th century, and one may wonder why. In 1763 Carl von Linné (1707–1778) published his book *Genera Morborum* in which he reintroduced the term to classify different 'species' of disease (e.g. morbi exanthematici (febrile diseases with spotted skin)).[10] Few were convinced of the wisdom of such a classification, and rather reiterated that the task of the doctor was in diagnosing the person – reopening the gulf between the Cnidian and the Coan philosophies.

The French, Bretonneau (1778–1862) and Laënnec (1781–1826) in particular, took up Linné's ideas of naming and classifying diseases, and started to match clinical phenomena with post-mortem findings. The diagnosis became a simple descriptive means to communicate a particular disease.[11]

Another way to understand the diagnosis is that of an explanation, describing and interpreting the patient's features. As Crookshank described it:

> ... diagnosis is just the first stage of the physician's work, the process of forming and expressing those judgments concerning the present state of the sick that guide us in our office of healing; and it consists in observation of the sick, interpretation of what is observed, and symbolisation of the interpretations accomplished.[11]

On the other hand, diagnosis can also be seen as a process, the ritual a doctor goes through to find particular features that match up with the images of past experiences, or academic memories.[11]

DISEASE: A DEFINITION

Despite all effort we have not created a unified framework defining disease. Even the widely used International Classification of Disease is a compromise, some sections being defined on an aetiological basis like infectious diseases, some on a pathophysiological basis like neoplasms or endocrine disorders, and some on an anatomical basis like cardiovascular or respiratory disesases.[10]

The disease concept is evolving constantly, and at times it is difficult to decide if new phenomena constitute disease. Rosenberg provides two examples that highlight this point:[9]

> . . . the American Psychiatric Association was undergoing an embarrassingly public struggle over the revision of its Diagnostic and Statistical Manual. Most conspicuously, psychiatrists voted, argued, then voted again as they reconsidered the problematic category of homosexuality. Was this a disease or a choice? How could a legitimate disease – in most physician's minds, a biopathological phenomenon with a characteristic mechanism and a predictable course – be decided by a vote, especially one influenced by feverish lobbying and public demonstrations.

> . . . at the end of the 20th century . . . we have become accustomed to seeing disease concepts being negotiated in public. On September 5, 1997, the *Philadelphia Daily News* reported that a school bus driver in rural Selinsgrove, Pennsylvania, felt, as he put it, like a woman trapped in a man's body and expressed himself by wearing women's clothing, a wig, and eyeliner while driving his bus to and from school. When anxious parents demanded that he be dismissed, the driver was perplexed: 'I don't understand what all the fuss is about. I am diagnosed with gender identity disorder syndrome, and I am being treated'.[9]

Another facet in the disease definition debate relates to the notion of normality, or rather abnormality.[12–14] Lowering the threshold at which a phenomenon now is regarded to be a disease has significant consequences – medical, psychological, social and economical.[8] Recent examples include the lowering of 'normal' cholesterol and 'normal' blood pressure readings result in up to 90% of the community having disease (*see* Figure 11.1).[15,16]

Technological ability is an additional source for disease generation; examples include mitral valve prolapse only seen on echocardiography, angina based solely on angiographic findings or peptic ulcer disease based on endoscopy appearance.

DISEASE: NOT AN OBJECTIVE STATE

The specifics of disease manifestations have taken the focus away from the human experience of illness.[17] Part of this human experience is shaped by our upbringing and by our social norms.[6] There is a large volume of literature showing the poor correlation of the objective disease state and clinical symptoms – or the illness experience; Baron cites the examples of peptic ulcer disease and diabetes, and comments that

> . . . by taking disease to be an anatomic or technologic fact, we are led further away from any ability to understand disease in human terms . . . our understanding of disease derives not from anything intuitive or anything the patient tells us, but rather from a reification of our model of the disease. Our understanding of the nature of disease is limited by

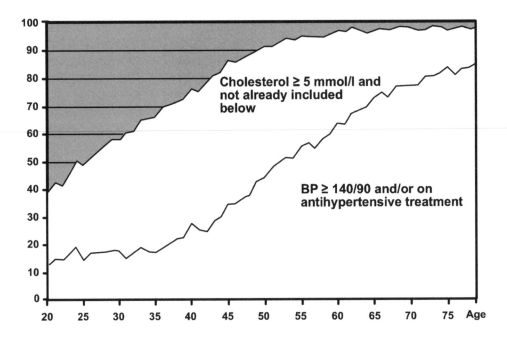

Figure 11.1 Point prevalence of individuals aged 20-79 years (men and women combined) with unfavourably high blood pressure (BP ≥140/90 mmHg) or cholesterol concentrations (cholesterol ≥5.0 mmol/l), as defined by the 2003 European guidelines on cardiovascular disease prevention in clinical practice. (Reproduced from Getz L, Kirkengen A, Hetlevik I, Romundstad S and Sigurdsson J. Ethical dilemmas arising from implementation of the European guidelines on cardiovascular disease prevention in clinical practice. A descriptive epidemiological study. *Scandinavian Journal of Primary Health Care*. 2004; 22: 2002-8,[16] with permission from Taylor and Francis AS.)

> our model, and entire aspects of the phenomenon of illness remain inaccessible or incomprehensible to us. We seem to have a great deal of difficulty taking seriously any human suffering that cannot be directly related to an anatomic or pathophysiologic derangement. It is as if this suffering had a value inferior to that associated with 'real disease' . . . In a sense, we seem obliged to remove ourselves from the world of our patients in order to categorize their diseases in a technologic manner.[17]

There is no doubt that our enhanced understanding of and ability to diagnose diseases has improved our disease management; however, the utility of our medical advances has to be balanced with our patients' needs.

> They derive their significance from what they mean for human beings and what effect they have on suffering and individual capability.[17]

The insight that disease is not an objective state but rather the product of our personal experiences led Fugelli to state

> That disease does not exist, only the experience of disease [does].[6]

DISEASE: BLURRING THE DISTINCTION, OR DISEASES WITHOUT EVIDENCE FOR DISEASE

An interesting phenomenon of the fascination with diseases is the *invention* of diseases for those in whom we cannot find 'disease', or put in a different way, where disease does not exist. Some call it non-disease,[18] some call it functional syndromes or somatisation,[19] and others call it psychosomatic disease. In reality we are dealing not with disease at all, but the physical representation of an illness experience.

ILLNESS

The illness and disease notions cannot be fully appreciated without being cognisant about historical and cultural aspects of those affected. Crookshank cites that

> ... throughout America, Indonesia and Papua-Melanesia; the notion that disease is an abstraction or loss of the soul, or vital principle, or a part thereof; in India and in Africa the belief that disease is due to a something added – a spirit or a demon. Clearly we have here a hint, and more, of the secular controversy between those who find in disease an impairment or failure of functional activity or adaptation – the Vitalists, who regard disease as an accident ... – and the Organicists, who explain all disease worth their attention in terms of physical attack on organs, and consider each described disease to be an entity ...[11]

Though we may construct our own illness in unique ways based on familial, ethnic and cultural beliefs, it is our experience of *feeling ill* that remains the driver for seeking medical – and at times lay or paramedical – care. Patients come to see us to *share* the story of their illness, to *make sense* of (or find meaning in) it, as well as getting relief from their symptoms. Are we prepared to listen, are we prepared to help them to understand their illness, or are we solely locked into the protocol of accumulating a series of facts, deciding upon a diagnosis and implementing a protocol-based treatment regimen? Are we Cnidians or Coans at heart?

Baron explored the differences in approach to patients in his paper 'An introduction to medical phenomenology: I can't hear you while I'm listening'.[17] Phenomenology stresses the careful description of phenomena in all their domains, and questions the erroneous beliefs inherent in the Cartesian dualism. Husserl strongly felt that the mind–body split prevents people from truly understanding themselves and the world around them, and he proposed to unite the abstract world of science with the concrete human world as it is experienced by the people.

Illness then, he argues, can be understood as a loss or disturbance of the *unconscious taking for granted of one's body*. As such, illness is a functional state, defined by the disruption of embodiment, rather than necessarily a structural change within one's body.

Understanding illness in this way, accepting that illness is intimately related to the patient's personality and his life experience, and understanding the doctor's role as helping patients to come to terms with, i.e. to find personal meaning in, their illness, has a profound impact on the way we organise and deliver health care. Illness is a whole person problem, not a problem of one part.[20,21]

Psychoneuroimmunology has shown that the whole-person effects of illness involve changes in immune-cell function leading to the 'subjective' signs of illness – symptoms of weakness, listlessness, changed sleep patterns, hyperalgesia and decrease in motivation and appetite.[22] Similarly 'objective' physical disease is associated with the same neuro-immunological changes.[23]

Being unable to separate the physical and the emotional components of the illness experience demands a systems rather than a mechanistic approach to the patient.[24] Thus an illness focus requires flexibility, and stands in stark contrast to the rigidity underlying principles embodied in evidence-based approaches to disease management, issues further explored later in this section.

HEALTH

Health is the proper relationship between the microcosm, which is man, and the macrocosm, which is the universe. Disease is a disruption of this relationship.

Dr Yeshi Donden, physician to the Dalai Lama

The balance notion is deeply anchored in the explanatory models of health and disease in many cultural traditions.[7] The philosophical ideas underlying health and disease are surprisingly similar, incorporating habitual, environmental and spiritual components, all of which acknowledge the complex interactions between the different aspects of human existence.

Pellegrino and Thomasma not only alluded to the inter-relationship of health and disease with the conception of medicine, but also emphasised the subjective and evaluative nature of these states:

> . . . the principal conception of medicine, health, and disease are necessarily related to, and acquire their meaning from, the epistemological features of clinical interaction. Both health and disease are essential conceptions of medicine as a discipline. To the objection that health and disease are definientia only of organ systems, one must counter with the large body of evidence that both concepts are evaluative; that is, they include in their meaning the values of patients, societies, and cultures.[7]

What then caused the crisis in confidence in the healthcare field in the latter half of the 20th century that led Taylor to conclude that

> . . . health is being portrayed as a state of continued negative reports for hidden disease.[25]

Viewed against this background it is not surprising then that the World Health Organization (WHO) and the World Organization of Family Doctors (WONCA) definitions of health struggle to include the subjective and evaluative dimension of health in their definitions:

... health is 'a state of complete physical, mental, and social well-being and not merely the absence of disease or infirmity'.[26]

... health is 'a state of optimal physical, mental, and social well-being and not merely the absence of disease or infirmity'.[27]

Nevertheless, around the same time Ivan Illich described health as a process that very much embraced the subjective and evaluative nature of health:

> The ability to adapt to changing environments, to growing up and to ageing, to healing when damaged, to suffering and to the peaceful expectation of death.[28]

SYSTEM MODELS OF HEALTH

As discussed earlier, health and disease were always seen in complex terms, and for the first time became effectively reduced to biomedical entities in the 20th century. This reductionist model did work well for defined disease states, but failed doctors and patient alike when the issue was one of a non-disease state. In 1977 Engel proposed a – still rather linear – complexity model, the biopsychosocial model of health, which was readily embraced especially by the primary care profession (*see* Figure 11.2).[29]

Parallel developments showed that the interactions between body parts occur by way of transmitters like hormones or electrical potentials. The material flow of hormones through the bloodstream, or of electrical potentials along a nerve or muscle, solely provide signals and do not equate to the content (or meaning) of the information transmitted. Its meaning arises from the overall functioning of the entire human organism, just as the phonemes of an utterance in a foreign language get their meaning only from the context of the speaker's language and way of life. The understanding of this distinction led Uexküll and Pauli to propose the need for biosemiotic thinking, meaning that one has to separate the interpretation of signals from the meaning assigned to them.[30]

In light of this Pauli *et al.* stated that:

> Contemporary science, by reducing all life phenomena to their physical or biochemical mechanisms, and their roles in communication to that of carriers of communication, profoundly limits the understanding of disease and even more so of health.[31]

By this criticism they did not mean to denigrate the achievements of the reductionist scientific method rather they argued one has to

> ... conceptualize health and disease as due in part not just to our material circumstances (e.g. genes and germs) but also to our life situations and the meanings we assign to these and other non-material circumstances.[31]

SYSTEMS HIERARCHY
(LEVELS OF ORGANIZATION)

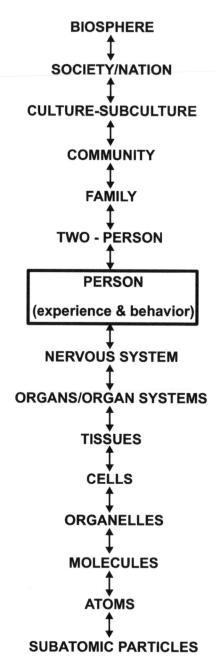

Figure 11.2 Biopsychosocial model of health. (Reproduced from Engel G. The clinical application of the biopsychosocial model. *American Journal of Psychiatry.* 1980; **137**: 535–44,[29] with permission from the American Psychiatric Association.)

HEALTH: A DYNAMIC STATE

One aspect in medicine has maintained stability, the notion of health being a balance between various aspects of a person's life experience and the need to make sense of, or find meaning in, the illness experience.

In conceptual terms, health (and disease) is neither solely an individual construction nor solely a reflection of societal attributes. The health experience has an objective as well as a subjective character. Individuals transform societal understanding of health by acting consciously, and social structures subconsciously influence the individual's health experiences.

This leads to the conclusion that health, illness and disease behave like complex adaptive systems. Health and illness need to be viewed simultaneously in terms of the somatic, psychological, social and semiotic dimensions. Health and illness affect the person at all levels of structures and functions.

Health viewed as a dynamic state reflects the levelled reality of the human experience. Figure 11.3 illustrates the somato-psycho-socio-semiotic model of health, describing health as a dynamically balanced state.[32,33]

In this model each corner represents one of the four domains of health and some of its characteristic elements. A strict delineation of each component is not possible as the domains are representational and symbolic in nature. Metaphorically, health is achieved when the individual perceives the forces exerted by each domain to be in balance. A patient's perception of balance may not equate to that of the physician, and may exist in the presence of disease and infirmity.[26,27] A qualitative study supports this latter point,

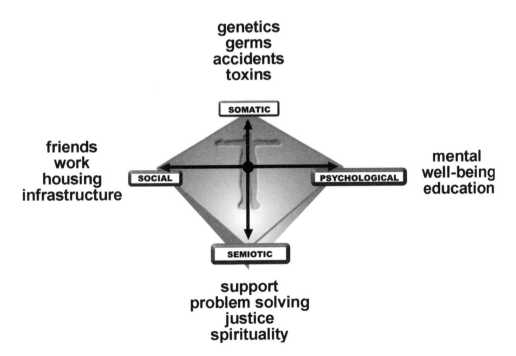

genetics
germs
accidents
toxins

friends
work
housing
infrastructure

mental
well-being
education

support
problem solving
justice
spirituality

Figure 11.3 The somato-psycho-socio-semiotic model of health.

99

**Shortness of Breath
EF 18%**

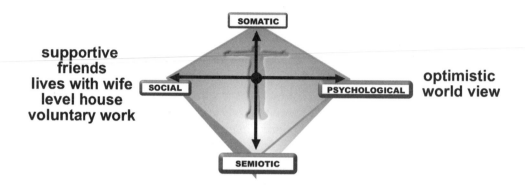

"I just happened to have had a heart attack"

**physically unfit
no chest signs or symptoms
EF > 50%**

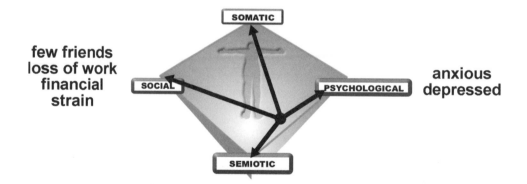

"Because I had a heart attack I now can't do a thing"

Figure 11.4   Health and an illness response. (EF = ejection fraction)

patients with knee osteoarthritis construct the need for total knee replacement in very different ways to justify their preferred treatment choice.[34]

The balance model incorporates the concepts of homeostasis – the body's ability to self-regulate to a position of stability and equilibrium in the face of challenge – and sense of coherence – the person's psychological adaptation and assimilation to challenges to his integrity.[35,36] Disturbance of this equilibrium leads to an illness experience, and we know that the direction of the disturbance or its severity lead to changes in all of the other domains. The examples in Figure 11.4 opposite show that the recognition of the inter-relationships between the domains in the somato-psycho-socio-semiotic model helps to achieve or work towards restoration of health – or healing – a point returned to in the next chapter.

SUMMARY POINTS

- Disease only exists after 'experts' have agreed that it exists as a clinicopathological phenomenon – a social construct.
- Disease exists if we can recognise it – a diagnosis.
- Disease exists as a deviation from the norm – a definition.
- Disease exists if we experience it or internalise the external social construct into our own personal construct – a personal experience.
- Illness is a the personal experience of being unwell/sick.
- Illness occurs in the presence and absence of disease.
- Health is not an ideal state – WHO/WONCA definitions.
- Health is an dynamic and evaluative state – a personal experience.
- A systems model of health integrates the fluid and personal disease and illness notions – the somato-psycho-socio-semiotic model of health.

SPECIAL ACKNOWLEDGEMENT

It is my great pleasure to thank Carmel Martin for her help with this chapter. Her vast knowledge and understanding of the health, illness and disease literature, coupled with her insights and critical review, greatly helped to substantiate the underpinnings of the somato-psycho-socio-semiotic model of health.

CHAPTER 12

The practice of medicine

Not medicines nor prescriptions heal, but trust.

Old Eastern wisdom

For a long time there has been a debate about medicine being a science or medicine being an art. Is it worthwhile to continue this debate, indeed, is there a need to make the distinction in the first instance? It would appear that such questions reflect the old Cartesian dualism of the reductionist paradigm. Ian McWhinney, in a discussion with the academic staff from the Department of General Practice at Monash University, Melbourne, Australia, put it this way:

> You could say that the whole question, 'Is it an art or is it a science?' is an old paradigm question, it's a question that arises from our dualistic view of the world where we like dividing things into two, and there was a quotation . . . this is actually from Whitehead but is quoted by one of his students, the American philosopher Susan Langer, what she says is that when an Epoch changes, or you could say, when a paradigm changes, it isn't that new answers are found to the old questions but that the old questions are just rejected, and the examples she gives [is] 'How was the world made?' and if you reply 'God made the world', that reply is in the same paradigm as the question. But if you reply 'The world wasn't made' then you reject the framework of the question and the paradigm, and the assumptions about the world, and conscious assumptions really determine the kind of questions we ask. So, I think, as things change some of the old questions will no longer be asked or no longer be seen to make sense, and the question 'Is it an art or is it a science?' will just become meaningless.[37]

CLINICAL KNOWLEDGE

One reason for this confusion arises from our understanding of knowledge in the clinical context. As has been shown in an earlier section worldviews are promulgated by belief systems at a particular time in history. Our Cartesian belief system goes back to the 17th century, has been reinforced by the science and technology successes of the 19th and 20th centuries, and has been further entrenched by Flexner's reforms of medical education. The net result for us as clinicians at the beginning of the new millenium is the unhappy state of being rooted in the sciences that fail us in the delivery of care to many individuals whose complaints do not have a science-based explanation (or disease in the biomedical sense).[2,24,38]

Given the social dimension of medical care we are often forced to pretend to have knowledge when the knowledge is incomplete or lacking, and we are often reluctant to confess and to stress the lack of what is known. Many issues turn out to be more complex than they appeared to be on first glance. As McCormick remarked:

> What is known defines the extent of the unknown, certainty the extent of uncertainty.[39]

In that environment clinicians have as much the task of understanding the patient as they have the task of understanding their diseases.[38] Both are ultimately contextual in nature.

Disease is believed to be objective – and probably is mostly so in the hand of the pathologist; however, diagnosing a disease is usually based on clinical and, to a lesser degree, on investigative data. These data are subject to observer judgements, and there is a large literature that has shown a high degree of interobserver variablity. Feinstein discusses these issues in great detail in relation to eliciting and interpreting clinical signs in his book *Clinical Judgement*;[40] the variability in the reporting of test results is equally well known, e.g. in mammography, radiography and histopathology.[41–43]

The different types of knowledge, and the world views and approaches to patients and their problems by different doctors are usefully depicted in the often-told joke about five doctors who went duck hunting.

> A general practitioner/family physician, a physician/internist, a psychiatrist, a surgeon and a pathologist go duck hunting. The general practitioner/family physician goes first, there are lots of ducks in the sky, he lifts his rifle, then puts it down and says, 'I think they are ducks, but I rather go for a second opinion'. Next time the ducks appear in the sky it's the physician's/internist's turn. He lifts his rifle just to put it down again and says to the other, 'I'm sure they are just common ducks, but just last night I read a review paper, and they commented that there is an endangered species that looks just like a common duck, so I really couldn't shoot them. Next is the psychiatrist. He doesn't even bother to lift his rifle and says, 'I know they are ducks, but do they?'. When the ducks appear again the surgeon lifts his rifle – bang, bang, bang . . . two dozen ducks fall out of the sky. When he is finished he turns to the pathologist and says, 'Go and see if they really were ducks'.

Clinical knowledge is contextual knowledge, and the context of this particular patient is best elicited and understood through the patient narrative. The particulars of this patient's problem become understandable, and the final treatment option is one that fits best with the patient's illness experience and expectations. Such an approach stands in stark contrast to a management strategy and guidelines based largely on available biomedical data.[24,38]

Clinical knowledge consists of some factual knowledge, a large component of personal knowledge gained from experience and reflection over time, and tacit knowledge, knowledge that cannot readily be made explicit, however plays an important role in dealing with the unique individual situation of a particular patient.[38] The following excerpt from Cochrane's autobiography may illustrate this:

> Another event at Elsterhorst had a marked effect on me. The Germans dumped a young Soviet prisoner in my ward late one night. The ward was full, so I put him in my room as he was moribund and screaming and I did not want to wake the ward. I examined him. He had obvious gross bilateral cavitation and a severe pleural rub. I thought the latter was the cause of the pain and the screaming. I had no morphia, just aspirin, which had no effect. I felt desperate. I knew very little Russian then and there was no one in the ward who did. I finally instinctively sat down on the bed and took him in my arms, and the screaming stopped almost at once. He died peacefully in my arms a few hours later. It was not the pleurisy that caused the screaming but loneliness. It was a wonderful education about the care of the dying. I was ashamed of my misdiagnosis and kept the story secret.[44]

Understanding and knowing in medicine and health care is multidimensional as well as contextual, and no one 'science' can define the base of the profession. As Ross Upsuhr concluded

> ... medicine and health care are not in need of a single solid foundation, but can operate well in a dynamic emergent framework ... health is as much human aspiration as scientific fact.[45]

THE ULTIMATE AIM OF MEDICINE: HEALING

Healing is the ultimate aim of medicine. The notion that the doctor is a healer is invariably identified with charlatanism and quackery. However this belief requires reconsideration in light of experiences like the one shared by Eric Cassel from his residency years in his book *The Healer's Art*.[46]

> ... I had a midnight call from the psychiatric ward: an old woman was having difficulty breathing. I found the patient gasping for air, her skin blue from lack of oxygen; she had full-blown pulmonary edema (water in the lungs) resulting from a blood clot in her lung. I sent the nurse for the urgently needed oxygen and drugs, but in those days, because of staff shortages and inexorably slow or inoperative elevators, a critically ill patient on a psychiatric ward in Bellevue at midnight might just as well have been in the East River: the wait for the necessary equipment would be interminable. I stood at the bedside feeling impotent, but the old woman's face and her distress pleaded for help. So I began to talk calmly but incessantly, telling her why she had the tightness in her chest and explaining how the water would slowly recede from her lungs, after which her breathing would begin to ease bit by bit and she would gradually feel much better. To my utter

amazement that is precisely what happened. Not only did her fear subside (which would not have surprised me) but the noises in her chest disappeared under my stethoscope, giving objective evidence that the pulmonary edema was, in fact, subsiding. By the time the equipment came, things were already under control and the patient and I felt as though together we had licked the devil.

I was, of course, immensely relieved and pleased, but I didn't know what to make of it. Now, twenty years later, I understand much better what had taken place in the middle of that night. I had felt helpless because none of the things I identified with a doctor's job of curing the sick were available; I had none of the technology which, to me, was essential to being a good doctor. What I didn't know then was that desperation and fear had led me unknowingly to function as a healer, a role traditionally played by physicians as far back as Hippocrates.[46]

As Cassel points out, a patient's sickness has two components, the disease and the illness, and it is the doctor's task to address both of these simultaneously. The notion of healing is much more global. It involves taking into account the patient's illness experience, the patient's background, ethnicity and culture and the environment in which it occurs, and the meaning the patient ascribes to his illness. It also involves the physician exploring his or her own response to the patient and the illness, as well as the patient's response to the physician.

Curing diseases has become the catch phrase and the intellectual framework for medicine in the 20th century. However for most non-communicable diseases of our time – heart disease, stroke, cancer – there is no available cure, and the *healing function* of the doctor, i.e. caring for the patient, becomes much more important.

SHARED UNDERSTANDING

The role of the physician is twofold – to understand the disease, and to understand the patient. The most essential step in understanding the patient is the establishment of a personal relationship between patient and doctor – a personal and individual process that cannot be standardised.[47,48] The danger of undermining the therapeutic relationship arises from the quest for unnecessary precision and spurious objectivity based on redundant technological investigations.[47]

This is not to say that scientific knowledge and technologies have not helped in the treatment of patients, but ultimately it is clinical wisdom, or phronesis as Aristotle termed it,[6] which provides the basis for healing. Clinical wisdom is the product of experience in clinical practice over time, coupled with one's knowledge about oneself. Healing requires the application of clinical wisdom in the context of and the knowledge about this patient. The effects are clear; patients who feel cared for are healthier, and are healthier for longer, than those who just get treated for their disease.[46]

Shared understanding leads to shared understanding of the meaning behind the illness or disease. As Tudor Hart put it:

> . . . to use medical science, doctors and patients will both have to learn that diagnoses are not beasts in the jungle to be hunted but human stories within real lives to be understood, with a past and a future, and these agendas will have to converge.[49]

Medical phenomenology and narrative-based medicine are ways to listen to and to understand the disease and illness experience of our patients and to help them to find and share the meaning of that experience.[17,50] It requires, as a central task of medical practice, that we reconcile scientific understanding with human understanding, using the one to guide the other. These are the recurring themes of the history and the philosophy of medicine – *medicine as a caring discipline*.

The case study in Box 12.1 illustrates the complexities of healing, and highlights how the fundamental concepts discussed so far work in the real lifeworld.

BOX 12.1 Case study

Mr R was a 53-year-old Bulgarian who had lived in Australia for 28 years. He managed a large knitting mill in the industrial area adjacent to our clinic and came to see me because he had heard that I had an interest in occupational health and physical medicine. He was still working when he related the story of his industrial accident which had occurred some four months previously. He was emptying cartons and other waste material into a large dumpmaster bin. In order to maximise the amount of waste it could hold it was his habit to jump into the bin and force the waste to the bottom. While he was inside the bin the truck that removed it on a weekly basis pulled up and began lifting it as the first stage of a manoeuvre that involves tilting it and tipping its contents into the truck which mechanically churns it up prior to disposal. The driver of the truck did not hear Mr R's cries to stop and somehow Mr R managed to leap out of the bin onto the ground below. This was a distance of some three or four metres. He did this just a few moments before he and the bin's contents were about to be emptied into the truck. He sustained multiple bruises but no fractures and after a short stay in hospital he was discharged home and subsequently discharged from the care of the orthopaedic specialist. There were no fractures, and bruising usually takes a week to settle. As far as the orthopaedic surgeon was concerned, Mr R would soon be cured. Unfortunately the pains continued and in fact worsened. There was constant neck and back pain as well as pains in the ankles and knees, with new symptoms such as chest pain and dysphagia developing. Mr R became depressed, could not sleep, had nightmares, developed impotence. He had divorced his first wife and was now married to a 33-year-old woman with whom he had a three-year-old son. His employer noted diminished performance at work and threatened to terminate his services unless he took stock of himself and put in more effort. He had seen a number of doctors, including rheumatologists and orthopaedic surgeons and was told that there was no organic cause for his symptoms. Afraid of losing his job, his marriage and possibly his life, he felt the need to continue seeking an answer.

When I saw him his main complaint was the chest pain and dysphagia. Although all the other pains were still present I considered that they had been adequately investigated. The chest pain had two components, one was ischaemic in nature, the other musculoskeletal. An electrocardiogram (ECG) showed definite ischaemic changes and his cholesterol was 7.2 mmol/l. He still smoked 30–40 cigarettes a day. Endoscopy did not reveal a cause for the dysphagia. Adding the diagnosis of ischaemic heart disease to his lists of complaints did not help, but at least it provided some explanation for one symptom and provided an opportunity to set treatment goals.

During our discussions two recurring themes emerged. One was related to the vision he had of himself being crushed to death in the truck. This vision haunted him day and night. The other was of his father committing suicide in Bulgaria. He (the patient's father) was married to a much younger woman who took a lover after her husband became impotent. Both of these themes had to do with his own perceived destruction and death, as he imagined history was repeating itself. In a short time he had gone from being an active, hardworking man with a positive self-esteem to a physical and emotional wreck.

It was clear that although a number of symptomatic cures were possible the road to healing would be a long and difficult one. After explaining this to him I suggested that a combination of psychotherapy from a specialist as well as counselling, support and physical treatment from me might be an appropriate course of action.

I cannot say that this story had an entirely happy ending. He lost his job, sued the employer for negligence, suffered an infarct, his wife left him and subsequently returned and it took some three years for him to rebuild his life. The case however, illustrates that the issues involved in healing are many and complex.[37]

The remainder of this chapter explores how psychoneuroimmunology, technology and the push of evidence-based doctrine impact on the function of healing.

PSYCHONEUROIMMUNOLOGY

Patients have always known about the effect of psychological and social stresses on their health. Working as a medical student in the early hours of the morning in casualty departments taught me that lessons – many of the patients presenting with myocardial infarction claimed that they were only here because of *that stress two days ago*.

Psychoneuroimmunology has taken up these anecdotes as the basis for studying the link between life experiences and health. The concept of psychoneuroimmunology goes back to Solomon and Moos, who in 1964 published a conceptual paper on the link between emotion, immunity and disease.[51] The link between psychological factors and immune function is summarised as:

> The endocrine system serves as one central gateway for psychological influences on health; stress and depression can provoke the release of pituitary and adrenal hormones that have multiple effects on immune function. For example, social stressors can substantially elevate key stress hormones, including catecholamines and cortisol, and these hormones have multiple immunomodulatory effects on immune function. In addition, distressed individuals are more likely to have multiple health behaviors that put them at greater risk, including poorer sleep, a greater propensity for alcohol and drug abuse, poorer nutrition, and less exercise, and these health behaviors have immunological and endocrinological consequences.[52]

Boxes 12.2–12.5 summarise findings from psychoneuroimmunology research that are of importance to general practice/family medicine and primary care; Box 12.2 lists a number of common life events associated with poorer immune function, Box 12.3 compares the difference in psychological wellbeing with immune function, Box 12.4 summarises the benefits of psychological intervention on the immune system and Box 12.5 lists the health consequences of stressful life events.

BOX 12.2 Common life events, particularly when associated with loss of control, lead to poorer immune function

- Caring for a dementing relative
- Job strain
- Burnout at work
- Unemployment
- Hurricanes and earthquakes
- Living near a damaged nuclear reactor

BOX 12.3 Psychological status and immune function

Negative mood:
- loss of sense of coherence
- relationship problems
- chronically abrasive or stressful personal relationships
- lack of social support
- depression

all lead to:
- decrease in natural killer cells
- increased rate of viral infection.

Optimism:
- is associated with slower progression of disease and prolonged survival in an HIV-positive patients
- gives a sense of coherence
- moderates immune response in association with anticipation of moving in the elderly

---

BOX 12.4 Benefits of psychological interventions on immune function

- Hypnosis
- Relaxation
- Classical conditioning
- Self-disclosure
- Those getting emotionally and cognitively involved in the disclosure process reorganise the meaning of the traumatic event and reduce avoidance of the stressful topic
- Exposure to a phobic stressor to enhance perceived coping self-efficacy
- Cognitive–behavioural therapies
- Improved immune function
- Reduced distress with traumatic events

BOX 12.5 Health consequences of stressful life events

- Poorer seroconversion to hepatitis, pneumococcal and influenza vaccines in the elderly, rubella in women of child-bearing age
- Higher risk of devolping a cold and influenza
- Cancer patients who did not participate in a stress reduction programme showed a faster progression of their disease, and a higher mortality rate
- Poorer wound healing
- Such events are likely to increase symptoms and progression in patients with autoimmune diseases and major depression

---

It is beyond the scope of this book to detail the mechanisms underlying the stress and immunoresponse in any detail, and interested readers are referred to Kiecolt-Glaser's work.[52]

THE ROLE OF TECHNOLOGY

Much of the known technology in medicine has been introduced since the Second World War. These technologies have significantly altered the way we perceive and perform medical care.[6,25,39,53] The influence of science and technology has been so pervasive as to achieve the belief that *all* human ailments can be overcome, and the faith in science and technology – held both by doctors and patients – has challenged the need for accepting suffering disease and illness.[6,53]

However many of the so-called breakthrough technologies have either been shown to be futile, or their utility in clinical care has never seriously been investigated.[25,54] In addition the over-reliance on technology risks the loss of trust in one's clinical abilities and judgements,[53] and thus tends to further erode the doctor–patient relationship, an issue we will return to in the next chapter.

ACCEPTANCE OF TECHNOLOGY

Technology has long played an essential part in human development, nevertheless we have had an ambivalent relationship with it.[47] As Feinstein put it:

> From the most ancient civilizations to the modern, the recorded attitudes about the ethical consequences of technologic advance indicate that man has been alarmed but assimilating, concerned but consuming.[40]

The introduction of the stethoscope by Laënnec in the 1830s examplifies this. The stethoscope was greated with great scepticism; in 1834, the *London Times* wrote:

> That it will ever come into general use notwithstanding its value . . . [is] extremely doubtful, because its beneficial application requires much time and gives a good bit of trouble both to the patient and the practitioner; because its hue and character are foreign, and opposed to all our habits and associations . . . There is something even ludicrous

in the picture of a grave physician proudly listening through a long tube applied to the patient's thorax. (cited in reference 40)

Today the stethoscope not only is commonplace, but is also a powerful symbol of the 'magic powers' of the doctor, closing the sequence of rejection, acceptance, abuse, regulation and incorporation of any new technology.[40]

ETHICAL DILEMMAS OF TECHNOLOGY

Besides the possibilities opened by technological advances, most technologies have not been fully evaluated in terms of their utility. We not only have saved lives with a particular invention, we also have caused many fatalities with the same.[40,53] How are we going to deal with these ethical dilemmas?

> . . . we have saved lives with blood transfusion, but have brought death to mismatched recipients; we have given the blessings of anaesthesia to patients undergoing surgery, but we have killed or paralyzed many with untoward reactions to anaesthetics; we have prevented the ravages of bacteria by using antibiotics correctly, but we have produced fatal or protracted illness with their abuse; we have made birth easier for the mother, but have injured the child removed untimely from its womb; we have learned to operate successfully upon every part of the human body, but we are not yet sure about when to do so, and in whom. Will clinicians of the future share our infatuation for the technology that makes possible these glories – and these tragedies? Will our clinical successors maintain the scientific urge to 'do something' that makes us so often ignore the clinician's sacred law of technologic regulation: primum non nocere?[40]

Besides our – the doctors' – fascination with technological possibilities, the cultural, and in particular the medicolegal, environment in many Western countries and the *un-realistic* expectations for nothing less than perpetual perfect outcomes, have dramatically increased the use of all technologies, not for their utilitiy, but for defensive reasons.

The belief that more interventions are safer though frequently clouds the reality of the real risk of doing harm.[12] This is illustrated in a comparative study of patients in two US states with a significantly different utilisation rate of angiography following myocardial infarction. Patients in one state had a 50% higher post-myocardial infarction angiography rate; however, patients in both states had the same rate of left main or three-vessel disease. The state with the higher angiography rate had a 50% higher coronary intervention rate (coronary artery bypass grafts or angioplasty), without any difference in immediate post-intervention mortality. Yet after two years of follow-up, the mortality risk was higher, and health-related quality of life was worse in the higher intervention state with a 40% higher angina and a 60% higher exercise intolerance rate.[55]

CLINICAL DECISION MAKING

In addition, the ready availability of technologies in Western healthcare systems has altered, or more precisely diminished, our clinical approach to and our clinical skills with patients.[47,53,56] History taking has become brief, physical examination has become limited, and clinical reasoning as a means to achieving a diagnosis is replaced by glancing over test results.[40,53] In the 1940s Harrison cited these changes to clinical care in his textbook as

> . . . the present-day tendency towards a five-minute history [is] followed by a five-day barrage of special tests in the hope that the diagnostic rabbit may suddenly emerge from the laboratory test.[57]

Today these changes to *patients' complaints* are most obvious in the area of neurological symptoms, where almost every patient will have a computerised axial tomography (CAT) scan or MRI as a matter of cause rather than as a matter of clinical evidence.[53] The influence of technology on clinical behaviour goes back at least a century, and appears to have its origins in the US. In 1912 a visiting French physician

> . . . reported his surprise at the number of laboratory tests routinely requested for the patients. To him the tests seemed 'like the Lord's rain, to descend from Heaven on the just and on the unjust in the most impartial fashion,' and he concluded 'that the diagnosis and treatment of a given patient depended more on the result of these various tests than on the symptoms present in the case.'[53]

The consequences of *relying* on technology-based data in our clinical practice are two-fold. In general we lose our *clinical skills* and our *human touch*, and in particular we redefine in our minds *complaints* into diseases based on technical data. The latter aspect is particularly concerning in primary care; as has been shown earlier the epidemiology of illness may vary, the epidemiology of disease however is rather static.[4]

Technology is a tool belonging to the Cnidian tradition of medicine – the influence of technology has changed our language and our thinking about patients, their illnesses and their illness experiences. The influence of technology has perpetuated the dehumanisation of the medical encounter.

TECHNOLOGY AND INTERFERENCE WITH HEALING

At this point the *psychological effects of technology on the physcian* as a means of overcoming his *discomfort with the uncertainties* underlying most illness presentations should be emphasised.[53] The perception of precision, standardisation and objectivity in part explains our belief in the reassurance of technology.[47]

Our perception of comfort and confidence are both qualities we largely gained in our formative years. For most of us these experiences occur(red) in the learning environment of the tertiary university hospital where the prevalence of unusual diseases is high, and where the successful diagnosis of these is often dependent on technology – we became converts. We are taking these experiences into community practice where technology is much less effective, and we fail to appreciate community epidemiology as the denominator for detecting disease.[53]

The instrumental success of technology in medicine has allowed us to cure many otherwise life-threatening diseases and to ease pain and suffering. However these advances have come at a price, with:

> ... medicine [being] accused of being cold, inhuman and addictive. Technological medicine is running up against its own limits. This, I believe, is because benefits and side-effects of medical intervention are of the same root; they both stem from technological objectivation of diseases. This objectivation leads on the one hand to effective intervention, but on the other hand to a technological bypass of communication.[54]

The shift to objectivation by technology has transformed the thinking and expectations of our patients.[54] They place more value on the data generated by technological investigations, regardless of the reassurances and explanations by their doctor.

> All the average patient in a consultant's office wants today is tests and plenty of them; he wants to 'be given the works'.[53]

Some do believe that a result must confirm their state of (physical) health and are reassured by this, for many the negative test results become an obstacle to their healing.[58] Technology has devalued the personal and therapeutic relationship with their physician.[47]

The significance of this phenomenon in relation to clinical practice has been explored by Daly and McDonald in the context of echocardiography.[58] A normal test did not automatically reasure the patient, and even though good doctor–patient communication was helping to resolve residual anxiety following a normal test, it was not predictably resolving these for every patient.

They also confirmed an old dictum that history and clinical examination alone *establish* a diagnosis in 83% of all patients. On the other hand, laboratory tests only helped to reach a diagnosis in 17% of cases where the clinician was unable to reach *any* diagnositc impression.[59] Not surprisingly Daly and McDonald could demonstrate that the doctor being confident in his clinical judgement about the normality of a patient's heart was accurate in all cases, thus echocardiography did not add anything to clarify the presenting problem, but maintained some patients' impaired health experience.[58] Figure 12.1 illustrates the effects of the science and technology lens on the functioning and the outcomes of the consultation.

THE ROLE OF EVIDENCE-BASED MEDICINE

Chapter 7 dealt with the underlying assumptions of science. Popper highlighted the fact that *all observations are always subjective*, and hence that only genuine and risky experiments that fail to falsify a hypothesis should be regarded as supporting. Kuhn stressed that in reality scientists usually work to verify their theories without questioning the underlying assumptions of their framework. Polanyi reinforced this point of subjectivity and underlying assumptions in science, stating

> For, as human beings, we must inevitably see the universe from a centre lying within ourselves and speak about it in terms of a human language shaped by the exigencies of human intercourse. Any attempt rigorously to eliminate our human perspective from our picture of the world must lead to absurdity.[57]

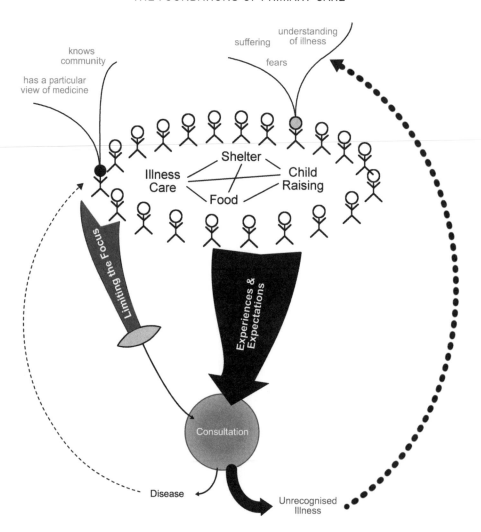

Figure 12.1   The effects of the doctor's science and technology lens on the consultation.

How do these notions fit with the call for practising evidence-based medicine (EBM), and the suggestion that we have *objective* knowledge about the subject matters in clinical care?

The debate about EBM is fierce at times. Despite their persuasive arguments and the backing of many institutions, governments and the legal system, the proponents of EBM have largely failed to convince clinicians, especially those working in primary care, to adopt their approach.[45] It is not because of clinicians denying the logic of using evidence, rather for the fact that the provided – rather *narrow, reductionist and population-based* – evidence appears rarely if ever to fit the complexities of the *individual patient* in front of them.[45,56,60]

COCHRANE'S APPROACH

Cochrane was driven by his desire for the NHS to be effective and efficient. He saw many flaws in the way governments of the day decided what treatments to provide for free. To overcome the biases inherent in the decision-making processes he proposed the vigorous use of the randomised controlled trial (RCT), stipulating very clearly that patients should be randomly selected from the *general population*.[61]

The basic principles of the randomised controlled trial

Rather than identifying personal characteristics in a population that contribute to a particular disease – the classical epidemiological study – the basic idea behind the RCT is not to worry about personal characteristics, but rather to select people blindly – or independent of the observer – into two equal groups. It is assumed that the characteristics of the people in each group are the same, and that one thus legitimately can test if one treatment is better than another. Results are then expressed as the observed difference *between the two populations* having or not having occurred due to chance (the famous *P* or probability value).[61]

Most in the medical profession hold the view that the RCT provides the only 'scientifically valid' evidence for clinical practice, a view derived from the influence of the statisticians.[62]

Most RCTs are intended to demonstrate the *safety* and *efficacy* of discrete clinical interventions,[12] e.g. using streptokinase in acute myocardial infarction,[63] lowering of blood pressure to prevent strokes, or screening mammography to prevent breast cancer death. Thus the comparisons only tell us – given that the intervention is effective – which of the two is more *efficient*, on a *population*, but not on an *individual*, level.[56] But as clinicians we are always dealing with that *one unique person* in front of us to whom we should apply *population evidence*.

> RCTs . . . are excellent at establishing group norms and common causality, but they fail absolutely in accounting for individual exceptions. Yet these individual exceptions are our patients, the people to whom we must apply this general knowledge.[64]

EVIDENCE-BASED MEDICINE IN PERSPECTIVE

Evidence is an undisputed a priori to clinical decision making.[62] Thus the definition of evidence-based medicine being:

> . . . the conscientious, explicit and judicious use of current best evidence in making decisions about the care of individual patients[65]

must be seen as a motherhood statement. This definition leaves wide open what should be regarded as evidence. In Warrell's words, it is necessary to ask the question

> . . . but what counts as best evidence? How persuasive are different kinds of evidence (or rather how persuasive ought they to be)? What happens when different kinds of evidence

point in opposite directions? What evidential role, if any, is played by 'clinical experience' or 'clinical expertise'? EBM needs a fully coherent, articulated and detailed account of the correct relationship between the evidence and various therapeutic and causal claims that would answer questions such as these from general first principles.[62]

Furthermore as the EBM proponents themselves pointed out, their belief of the superiority of their method cannot be substantiated.

> The proof of the pudding of evidence-based medicine lies in whether patients cared for in this fashion enjoy better health. This proof is no more achievable for the new paradigm than it is for the old, for no long term randomized trials of traditional and evidence-based medicine are likely to be carried out.[66]

In this context the criticisms voiced against EBM are hard to deflect – EBM being narrow and reductionist,[56] ignores clinical judgement and expertise, inappropriately relies on epidemiology[60] and statistics, dogmatically adheres to the randomised controlled trial, neglects the different ways physcians and healthcare workers know,[67] is uncertain what to regard as evidence in the first place,[68] views values as opposites to evidence, ignores the existence of the grey areas in clincial practice,[69] and so forth.

THE RANDOMISED CLINICAL TRIAL IN PERSPECTIVE

The first major concern about RCTs is the selection of patients. Britton reviewed the literature and found that many studies had too narrow inclusion criteria, those at high risk of adverse effects and those believed to have a relatively small or no benefit or those believed to be lost to follow-up being excluded; many blanketly excluded the elderly, women and ethnic minorities without providing a rationale, and most patients were selected from university hospital environments. Consequently patients in intervention trials generally are more seriously ill, and tend to have a different prognosis than patients identified from clinical databases. Patients participating in prevention trials are more likely to already have adopted healthier lifestyles than non-participants. All of these factors tend to overexaggerate the benefits of intervention, and underestimate the benefits of prevention trials.[70]

A second concern is the overestimation of the benefits of a particular treatment during a trial when compared to the benefits observed after introduction into routine practice. Lauritzen *et al.* showed that on the one hand patients allocated to the control group improve their *health* simply by participating in a trial without altering their objective disease control (Hawthorne effect), and on the other that patients in the study group who continued their treatment in routine clinical care after the trial period lose much of the improvement in their objective disease control (*see* Figure 12.2).[71]

RCTs are widely believed to be the 'gold standard' of medical research evidence. However Concato *et al.* did find '*no good evidence*' to support that notion,[72] and in fact the results of RCTs on the same condition show much more heterogeneous and at times contradicting outcomes then well-designed observational studies on the same subject.

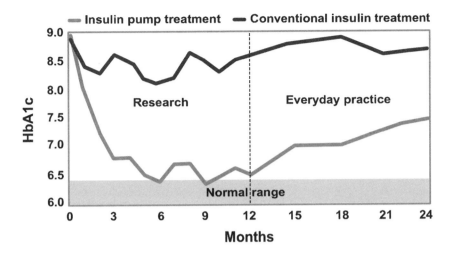

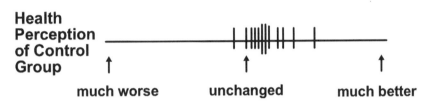

Figure 12.2   Trial and everyday practice. The intervention group improved their disease control significantly, however much of this improvement was lost after reverting to everyday practice (top). However the health experience of those in the control group (Hawthorne effect) also improved significantly (bottom). (Reproduced from Lauritzen T, Mainz J and Lassen J. From science to everyday clinical practice. Need for systematic evaluation of research findings. *Scandinavian Journal of Primary Health Care.* 1999; **17**: 6-10,[71] with permission from Taylor and Francis AS.)

Our results challenge the current consensus about a hierarchy of study designs in clinical research. Contrary to prevailing beliefs, the 'average results' from well-designed observational studies (with a cohort or case–control design) did not systematically overestimate the magnitude of the associations between exposure and outcome as compared with the results of randomized controlled trials of the same topic. Rather, the summary results of randomized, controlled trials and observational studies were remarkably similar . . . Viewed individually, the observational studies had less variability in point estimates (i.e. less heterogeneity of results) than randomized controlled trials on the same topic. In fact, only among randomized controlled trials did some studies report results in a direction opposite that of the pooled point estimate, representing a paradoxical finding.[72]

Part of the problem of these findings may well be attributable to the design and the conduct of a RCT, despite its described rigorous approach.

The treatment effects were most similar when the exclusion criteria were similar and when the prognostic factors were accounted for in observational studies.[70]

Most RCTs are intended to demonstrate the safety and efficacy of discrete clinical interventions, and occasionally they provide evidence of harm (when the false positive rate is higher than true positive rate):[12]

> Mindless investigation is almost as common as mindless prescribing. There seems to be little general awareness of the effect of the prevalence of disorders on positive predictive value. Even with highly specific tests when the prior probability of abnormality is low, false positives far outweigh true positives, a major problem in screening procedures.[39]
>
> Medicine in meeting the needs of patients, and the needs of doctors, assumes the mantle of wisdom, authority, and power. There is little room for confessions of ignorance or therapeutic pessimism. Pressures toward activism arise in part from our patients, but the assumption that patients require something to be done also provides a convenient rationalization for meeting our own needs. A stroke in the untreated borderline hypertensive is medical failure; in the treated, it is an act of God.[39]

The final and potentially most serious concern is a conceptual one.[60,62] The RCT 'is [wrongly] seen' as demonstrating a cause and effect relationship in the Newtonian reductionist sense. This assumption is untenable on many grounds, not least the observations from studying the placebo effect and psychoneuroimmunology research, both showing that other pathways are highly influential in determining the intended outcome over and above that exerted by the intervention.

INTERPRETING RESULTS

Statistical numbers are frequently abused, and commonly not well understood among clinicians, and how easily clinicians can be misled on the basis of quoting a 'big number' is illustrated in Figure 12.3.[54,56] Many studies do not report the prevalence of the condition in the community, and instead use relative risk reduction (RR) as the number to justify the introduction of change to clinical practice, without considering the absolute risk reduction (AR) – or the number needed to treat (NNT) – for one benefit to occur, which in fact may be very small.

> Common sense, regardless of scientific training, would appreciate that relative risk is no basis for modifying behavior unless absolute risk is appreciable. When absolute risks are small, small increases in relative risk are of no practical importance. Yet on the basis of data of this kind, we have induced neuroticism and hypochondriasis on an unprecedented scale.[39]

Recently it was suggested to not only provide figures that indicate the positive impact of an intervention (AR reduction or NNT), but also those that indicate how many would not benefit – the number treated needlessly (NTN).[73] Mathematically, NTN = NNT – 1; from Figure 12.3 the best case scenario of NNT = 100, NTN = 99, or expressed as a ratio – the index of therapeutic impotence (ITI) – ITI = 99%, a stark reminder of our interventional and therapeutic limitations.

It must become an ethical imperative to educate all in these basic statistical concepts, and to unequivocally rebuke those who try to misuse them for ulterior motives. It also must translate into clinical practice in terms of truly discharging our *informed consent* obligations, and allowing patients to forego potential small benefits in light of the extra burden placed on them by interventions.[73]

A related issue is that of *biased reporting of study results in medical journals*. McCormack and Greenhalgh illustrate this issue in relation to the UK prospective diabetes study (UKPDS) which has been widely reported as 'demonstrating the benefits of tight glucose control as the key to improving outcomes'. However the results are less clear – sulphonylureas and insulin did not prevent macrovascular endpoints, however, metformin did, and did so somewhat independently of the reduction in blood sugar control.[74]

THE DIFFERENT WAYS OF KNOWING

Chapter 7 explored the notion of knowledge in detail. Here it should be reiterated that there is more than one way of knowing, and this critical stance towards EBM reflects the discomfort with the implied notion that only *hard evidence* is worth considering seriously.[56] The underlying assumption of the RCT that randomisation creates two equal groups to demonstrate effectiveness, rather than efficency, is fundamentally flawed.

Rather more intriguing questions arise: if one treatment is better than another, why does that treatment not work for all? How do patients who do not benefit from a treatment differ from those who do, and how can a large proportion of patients achieve the same outcome from no intervention? How can we identify responders and how can we help those who failed to respond to an 'effective' treatment?

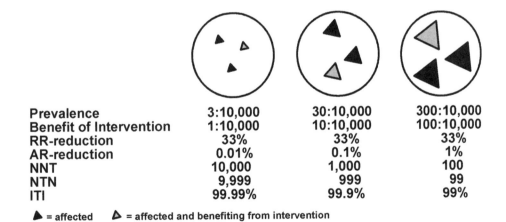

Prevalence	3:10,000	30:10,000	300:10,000
Benefit of Intervention	1:10,000	10:10,000	100:10,000
RR-reduction	33%	33%	33%
AR-reduction	0.01%	0.1%	1%
NNT	10,000	1,000	100
NTN	9,999	999	99
ITI	99.99%	99.9%	99%

▲ = affected △ = affected and benefiting from intervention

Figure 12.3   Interpreting evidence in context. Statistically relative risk reduction is independent of and absolute risk reduction is dependent on the prevalence of the condition under study. Even a 1% absolute risk reduction will mean 99% of patients receiving a particular intervention will have no benefit at all. See text for explanation of abbreviations.

The RCT has its place in medical research; however, it is limited to the small number of problems that are very well but narrowly defined, where the intervention is very specific, and the observation period short, like the use of streptokinase in acute myocardial infarction on mortality within 28 days.[63] Long-term studies using randomisation are no different from any other prospective observational study. Having focused on one variable only, they fail to consider other factors besides the intended intervention, as possible explanations for the observed outcomes, i.e. for both those who benefited and those who did not.

SUMMARY POINTS

- Belief systems and world views influence how we 'as doctors' see/perceive the patient's complaint.
- Doctors are healers, healers of illness and where possible disease.
- The personal relationship between the doctor and the patient is the foundation of the healing relationship.
- Clinical wisdom, or phronesis in Aristotle's terms, provides the basis for healing.
- The patient's narrative provides the basis for achieving a shared understanding of the illness.
- Psychoneuroimmunology has demonstrated the neuroendocrine changes associated with illness and healing.
- Technology has provided some improved precision in the diagnostic process.
- Many technology-based interventions have failed to improve the patient's health, and in fact have substantially decreased morbidity and increased mortality.
- Technology-based interventions frequently fail to alleviate the patient's anxieties, thus interfering with the healing process.
- RCTs have by necessity decontextualised the somato-psycho-socio-semiotic world of the individual patient.
- RCTs provide information about the efficiency of treating a specific population, assuming that interventions are highly specific and associated with linear outcomes.
- Reporting relative improvements of outcomes between two approaches over-represents the true benefit.
- Most RCTs demonstrate negligible clinical improvements in outcomes.

CHAPTER 13

Practising general practice/family medicine

> If you see something from a distance, and you do not understand what it is, you will be content with defining it as an animal, even if you do not know whether it is a horse or an ass. And when it is still closer you will be able to say it is a horse, even if you do not yet know its name. Only when you are at the proper distance will you see that it is Brucellus, the abbot's horse, and that will be full knowledge, the learning of the singular.
>
> *Umberto Eco* – The Name of the Rose

General practice/family medicine operates in the community, characterised by a high prevalence of illness and a low prevalence of disease.[3,4] Many presentations occur at the early clinical stages of the ailment, making it impossible to decide with any degree of certainty about the true nature of the problem. Figure 13.1 illustrates the working environment of general practice/family medicine, and some of the important factors impacting on the clinical decision-making process.

THE PERSON AT THE CENTRE OF MEDICAL CARE
COMMITMENT TO THE PERSON
General practice/family medicine is characterised by its commitment to the person, rather than a specific disease, technology, sex or age group.[20] We are committed to the patient because of the experience of *illness*, regardless whether its cause is medical or non-medical.[20] Illness is a problem of the whole person, and not a problem of a particular part,[20] or to paraphrase Osler, the person is more important than his illness. The following excerpt from Baron's paper illustrates this point, and it should remind us how easy it is to forget to enquire about the consequences of a diagnosis on the patient:

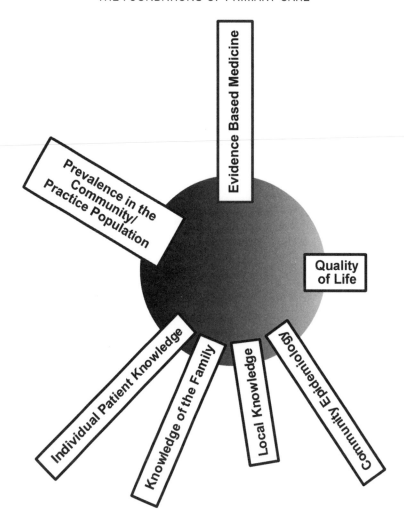

Figure 13.1 Factors impacting on clinical decision-making in general practice/family medicine.

I have long been a potter, a bachelor, and a leper. Leprosy is not exactly what I have, but what in the Bible is called leprosy (see Leviticus 13, Exodus 4:6, Luke 5:12–13) was probably this thing, which has a twisty Greek name it pains me to write. The form of the disease is as follows: spots, plaques, and avalanches of excess skin, manufactured by the dermis through some trifling but persistent error in its metabolic instructions, expand and slowly migrate across the body like lichen on a tombstone. I am silvery, scaly. Puddles of flakes form wherever I rest my flesh. Each morning I vacuum my bed. My torture is skin deep: there is no pain, not even itching; we lepers live a long time, and are ironically healthy in other respects. Lusty, though we are loathsome to love. Keen-sighted, though we hate to look upon ourselves. The name of the disease, spiritually speaking, is Humiliation.

> If you read this and said, 'Aha! I know what this man has: psoriasis!', you should ask
> yourself why you rejected the patient's own diagnosis – humiliation. The vivid contrast
> between the medical understanding of his disease ('some trifling but persistent error in
> its metabolic instructions') and the patient's understanding ('torture . . . ironically healthy
> . . . loathsome . . . Humiliation') is arresting. From the first paragraph of this story, we are
> confronted with the poverty of medical description.[17]

Two factors determine the degree of understanding the patient – the ongoing relationship
with the patient over time,[75] and the intimacy of the doctor–patient interaction in the
consultation.[24][47] Both are required for the development of a trusting – and effective –
relationship.[76] The more we know the patient and the more we understand his particular
situation, the less likely we are to think about him in categorical disease terms. Our
task is to deal with his illness, including the disease component, rather than simply
approaching his problems by applying disease management guidelines.

UNDERSTANDING THE PERSON'S CONTEXT
Understanding the personal perspective of the patient alone is not sufficient for placing
the patient in the centre of medical care. Illness occurs in the context of the patient's
life circumstances – his family, friends, culture, work and so forth.[21] Knowing the local
community – its composition, its infrastructure, its tensions – are all essential parts
of truly understanding the patient. The health effects of local environments will be
explored further in more detail later.

THE KNOWLEDGE BASE OF GENERAL PRACTICE/FAMILY MEDICINE

The working knowledge of medicine at large, but general practice/family medicine in
particular, possesses three equal components – the factual knowledge about diseases, the
practical knowledge of the craft, and the personal knowledge of insight and awareness.[20]
An understanding of the importance of the patient's experience of health and illness is
an important aspect of our medical knowledge.[24]

All of these knowledge components allow us to effectively help patients to deal with
their illness experience: by providing an explanation describing the mechanisms behind
the illness; by attempting a cure even though we will never really achieve the same state
that was present prior to the onset of the illness; and by providing a prediction, helping
patients to plan for the future.[17]

Figure 13.2 illustrates the knowledge domains of general practice/family medicine
adopting the Cynefin (Welsh; pronounced kun-ev'in) approach, a method that highlights
the different level of complexity inherent in potential patient presentations, all of which
may well be applicable at a certain point in time.[77] Consultations dealing with the
common, acute, non-life-threatening and stable chronic illnesses require solid textbook
knowledge, whereas acute, life-threatening, unstable chronic and psycho-socio-semiotic
illnesses also require tacit knowledge and intuition associated with the ability to detect
linkages between a variety of contributing, but not necessarily causative, variables.

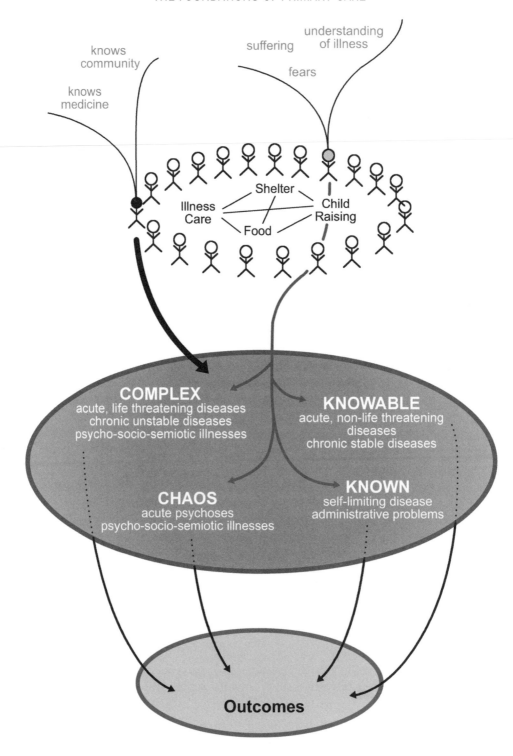

Figure 13.2 The knowledge domains of general practice/family medicine.

CONSULTATIONS IN GENERAL PRACTICE/FAMILY MEDICINE

White and Green outlined the epidemiology of illness in the community demonstrating that illness is common, but somehow only one-third of those feeling ill are seeking medical care.[3,4] Kleinman described the process of becoming a patient as

> ... typically lay people activate their health care by deciding when and whom to consult, whether or not to comply, when to switch between treatment alternatives, whether care is effective, and whether they are satisfied with its quality ... We can think of the following steps occurring, at least initially; perceiving and experiencing symptoms; labelling and valuating the disease; sanctioning a particular kind of sick role (acute, chronic, impaired, medical, or psychiatric, etc), deciding what to do and engaging in specific health care seeking behaviour; applying treatment; and evaluating the effect of self-treatment and therapy obtained from other sectors of the health care system. The sick person and his family utilise beliefs and values about illness that are part of the cognitive structure of the popular culture.[78]

Thus the physician must understand the disease as well as the patient.[47] Understanding the person in a holistic way means to embrace him as a complex adaptive system, with properties like growth, regeneration, healing, learning, self-organisation and self-transcendence.[24]

As such a person's illness cannot be understood in deterministic ways, we may have a 'good idea' how this illness may most likely behave; however, in the particular circumstances of this patient another outcome can be envisaged. General practice/family medicine is constantly dealing with *a particular circumstance* in a complex environment, thus always having to deal with a degree of uncertainty.[24]

Given that a living organism is in a constant state of a dynamic equilibrium, that all information reverberates through the system through feedback loops, the organism will respond in its entirety to a change to any part. Thus in a dynamic system the cause of an illness may be a trigger, yet the reason for not healing or responding to treatment may be quite different, and without identifying the latter one the patient will *maladapt* and end up with a continuing illness – often (inappropriately) referred to as chronic disease.

In complex adaptive systems, cause and effect are usually distant from each other; cause and effect are dependent on time and place, and usually an outcome is dependent on multiple processes, and any outcome in a particular instance is hard to estimate.[24] In technical terms it is easy to determine the relationships between events, but it is virtually impossible to attribute direct causality between them.

Being able to outline the relationships between events and resulting outcomes or consequences of these relationships facilitates the sense-making process, and leads to the discovery of the meaning behind the events.[21]

Meaning, emotions and memory are closely linked in the self-organising structure of the human system. Neuroendocrine studies have shown the influence of emotions and life experience on the immune system and life expectancy. There is also the evidence of social embeddedness and resistance to disease – social isolation increasing the morbidity of virtually every disease. Social factors are part of the interconnectedness of the person's system.

Hence bodily sensation is a reflection of mindful knowing of the world. Emotions are necessary for cognition and memory, and especially for giving meaning to our experiences. Neurosciences have demonstrated these connections being laid down in the structure of our brain, with important experiences, including their affective colouring, and their associated meaning to us, being 'hardwired' in our neural circuits. Our life events, our personal narratives, are stored in this way, giving us our sense of self, and enabling us to integrate and make sense of new experiences.[24]

General practice/family medicine is the only discipline that has the potential to overcome the Cartesian dualism of body and mind through its embrace of an understanding of the relationships and the interconnectedness of the whole system of the human being.[24]

Additionally general practice/family medicine, through its commitment to *personal doctoring*, remains the one stable place for patients in a rapidly and unpredictably changing social and medical world. The awareness of and the insights gained from being close to the community provide the opportunity to contribute to societal development.[79]

PERSONAL RELATIONSHIP WITH PATIENTS

Most patients who have access to primary care services develop a long-term relationship with *their* doctor. This personal relationship between the doctor and the patient is the most important building block of general practice/family medicine.[6,20,24,79] Ian McWhinney's affirmation

> To restore the primacy of the person, one needs a medicine that puts the person in all his wholeness in the center of the stage and does not separate the disease from the man, and the man from his environment – a medicine that makes technology firmly subservient to human values, and maintains a creative balance between generalist and specialist. These I believe to be the aims of family medicine[22]

not only has summarised the wisdom of doctoring over the past 3000 years but also provided us with the direction for the future at a time of general confusion about the role and goals of doctors and medicine in society.

The personal relationship transcends the patient's entire lifespan as well as the entire spectrum of ailments. Personal relationships develop from listening to patients' narratives of their illnesses over time, rather than being 'a waste of time' as many have perceived it;[53] it is the process of gaining the tacit knowledge needed when critical decisions have to be made, and evidence does not exist.[45,47,56]

PATIENT CENTREDNESS

Relationships define the discipline of general practice/family medicine,[7] and patient-centredness is the therapeutic mode of the consultation in general practice/family medicine. The patient-centred approach aims to understand the patient and his illness in context of his beliefs, family, culture, work and so forth, and is centred on the patient's narratives.[21,80]

In patient-centred medicine, the patient is a partner in the therapeutic relationship which has been shown to enhance self-healing, and directly connects with the Socratic philosophy discussed in Chapter 6. The benefit of patient-centredness is not only better communication but also improved emotional health, functional status, disease control and pain control.[80–83]

In addition patient-centred consultations achieve higher satisfaction of both the patient and the doctor, are on average shorter, and lead to reduced resource use – better compliance with medications, and fewer investigations and referrals.[80,84] It is of great importance to the health of our patients not to lose patient-centred care as a result of health reforms.[83]

TRUST

The first prerequisite to developing trust is an ongoing doctor–patient relationship combined with a patient-centred approach.[80,85,86] Developing trust requires time to listen to the patient's story and to gain insight into the patient's understanding of his condition – most doctors are not yet patient-centred and interrupt the patient's story after only 18 seconds.[80,81,86,87] Listening and trying to understand the patient's meaning of his illness is especially needed in times when technological investigations fail to provide any lead.[53]

Trust is the belief that the sincerity, benevolence and truthfulness of others can be relied on, and usually implies that the trusted person will act in one's best interest. Sharing the same beliefs fosters the development of trust between doctors and patients, as does the patient's perception that the doctor knows him well.[81,88] These are but two reasons why personal doctors are still trusted, even if many patients do not trust the healthcare system any more.[76] Being ill means being vulnerable; seeking medical care means entrusting one's recovery to the doctor,[5 74] and trust in the physician strongly relates to the outcomes of care.[7,76,88–90]

> Sick people have always had a particular need for trust, because to fall ill implies a loss of trust in yourself, in your body, in your social role, in your future. This loss of trust fortifies the need to trust others; among them, the doctor.[76]

PHRONESIS

The Aristotelian concept of phronesis refers to the notion of practical wisdom. Practical clinical wisdom is gained by experience in the context of the individual consultation.[6] It requires more than just arriving at a diagnosis, it requires personal insights, and it requires discourse between patient and doctor. Phronesis requires a commitment to oneself, being critical about one's knowledge, skills and performance, as much as it requires one's commitment to understanding the patient. The accelerating commercialisation and bureaucratisation of health care are major threats to practising medicine wisely; the new language has become the tool to threaten and to change our mental mindsets.[6,91]

Key words are: managed care, gate-keeping, fund holding, cost-effectiveness and quality control. Patients are redefined as units of production. Diagnosis and treatment are given a price. The profit of investing in treatment procedures is calculated in quality-adjusted life years.[6]

CONSULTATION LENGTH

Time is an important factor in the consultation. As has been discussed the doctor–patient relationship develops with time and over time, and with it, develops all important tacit knowledge and trust between the patient and his doctor. Longer consultations allow the discussion of psychosocial issues, are more comprehensive (more health promotion and prevention), and lead to higher satisfaction and higher enablement. Despite the perception that time is the most expensive resource in medicine, longer consultations are not only more effective but also associated with lower resource use.[49,92–97]

The population in most Western countries is ageing, and more patients present with several diseases concomitantly, increasing the demand for consultation time. For most of these health problems cures are not available, increasing the need to help patients to make sense of their failing health and the associated illness experience.

The increasing demand for more care and the increasing need for longer consultations coupled with the increasing worldwide shortage of primary care doctors threaten the very concept of personalised somato-psycho-socio-semiotic care, a threat that will be one of the greatest challenges to the concept of medicine at large. (*See* Figure 13.3.)

PROTECTING PATIENTS FROM 'MEDICAL EXPLOITATION'

The personal and ongoing relationship with patients provides general practitioners/ family physicians with a unique window into their patients' personal ways of dealing with their diseases and illnesses, and their way of handling the slow deterioration in health. This deep understanding of the individual allows general practitioners/family physicians to share the burden of the imperfection of life and medical care. It helps to advocate the human right for imperfection,and to allow the proper balancing between needed and doubtful intervention.[6]

The issue of protecting patients from unnecessary interventions is particularly pertinent when harm is potentially high. Common situations include those where the spectrum of disease does not impact on either a good or poor prognosis, where there is a competing risk of death from other causes even if a treatable disease is successfully treated, where the patient is not bothered by current symptoms and where the risk of treatment outweighs the potential benefits of treatment.[12]

CONTINUITY OF CARE

Continuity of care is one of the defining characteristics of general practice/family medicine and a consequence of the personal relationships with patients. The term goes back to the 1960s, and the first rigorous conceptualisation and exploration appeared in 1975 in a series of articles by Brian Hennen, Ian McWhinney, Marc Hansen and John

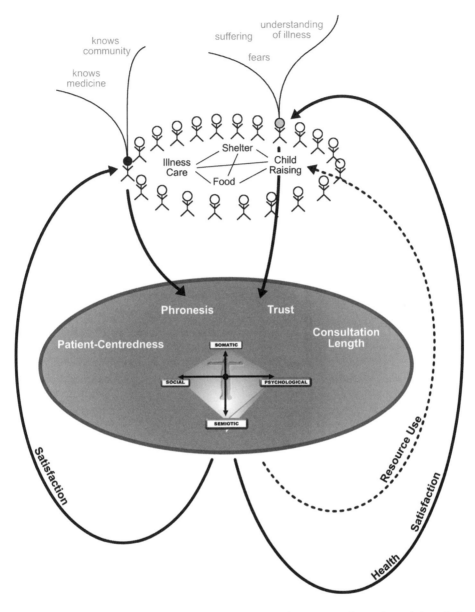

Figure 13.3 The general practice/family medicine approach. Patient-centredness, phronesis (practical wisdom), trust and consultation length are core attributes of the general practitioner/family physician consultation, and all contribute to improved patient satisfaction and health outcomes.

Geyman.[98–101] Since then, continuity of care has been studied extensively, but many questions about the concept and its impact on healthcare delivery and healthcare outcomes remain unanswered. Table 13.1 summaries the early conceptual work in terms of the different dimensions of continuity.

TABLE 13.1 The linear dimensions of continuity of care

DIMENSION	CHARACTERISTIC
Chronological[98]	The care of patients of all ages
	The change of health over time, change in the individual or change in the natural history of the illness
Geographical[98]	The place of care where the patient is seen – surgery, home, hospital or nursing home
	The place where the physician is available
Interdisciplinary[98]	The caring for multiple diseases in the same patient
	Dealing with the illness experience of the patient and his family
	Co-ordinating the management to restore the function of the whole family
Interpersonal[98]	The doctor–patient relationship
	Interpersonal family relationships
	The relationships with other healthcare professionals involved in the care of the patient
Informational[98,102]	The keeping of adequate medical records
	Good communication between doctors and other healthcare providers
Accessibility[102]	Convenient offices
	Effective appointment systems
	The provision of after-hours care
	Ease of access to medical advice
Stability[102]	The community
	The family and the individual
	The provider himself

Many issues discussed over time remain pertinent for the future development of primary care. Section 5 will deal with this issue in more detail; nonetheless, some important aspects should be highlighted at this point. Firstly, there is the notion, put forward by Becker and colleagues in 1974, who asserted that

> . . . the need to provide 'continuity of care' is a basic public health and medical care tenet
> . . . and a *sine qua non* to what is currently viewed as 'good' medical care.[103]

Hjortdahl defined continuity of care as a defining element of the discipline of general practice/family medicine (1990):

> A central element in this new specialty [i.e. general practice] is continuity of care – an orientation away from fragmentation of patient care and toward an integrated medical care model . . .[104]

Banahan and Banahan stressed the interpersonal relationship between doctor and patient from an attitudinal perspective (1981):

> Continuity of care is a phenomenon that occurs between a patient and physician, which can best be described as a contract. Since it is a contract involving attitudes, it will

be referred to as an attitudinal contract. Analysis of existing good physician–patient relationships reveals three essential characteristics of the attitudinal contract; (1) a beginning point, (2) an end point, and (3) quality.[105]

In 1989 McWhinney highlighted that continuity of care is more than simply an ongoing relationship, it entails the notion of commitment and responsibility for the patient:

> Continuity is not only a question of duration . . . Continuity in family practice is an unbroken responsibility to be available for any health problem through to the end, whatever course it may take.[106]

Hjortdahl recognised early the changes in the healthcare environment and the changing role of the primary care provider. The initial subtle changes over time have led to a crisis in confidence in their abilities:

> . . . as medicine is becoming increasingly complex, the image of the family physician as being the patient's sole doctor could be deemphasized. A major function could instead be that of having the overall knowledge and coordination responsibility for the different health needs of the patient.[104]

For Gonella and Herman, continuity of care must have a utility arising from the otherwise mechanistic aspect of an ongoing relationship (1980):

> [Continuity of care] is of value only to the extent that it has an impact on outcomes of care, the prevention or reduction of physical, mental, or social disabilities, the satisfaction of patients, and the costs of care.[107]

DEFINING CONTINUITY OF CARE

A recent literature review was not able to come up with a unifying definition of continuity of care, but highlighted that continuity involves the coherent and connected and consistent way of linking discrete healthcare events in a personal context over time, and suggested that there are three types of continuity in the healthcare setting – informational, managerial and relational.[108] Another review refers to a hierarchical model of continuity of care, the first level being informational, the second longitudinal and the third interpersonal.[109]

Continuity of care has multiple dimensions, the more we try to understand continuity, the more it becomes clear that it is a complex construct, adapting to change and opening space for new possibilities in clinical care. Not surprisingly practising general practitioners/family physicians have an acute awareness of these complexities, and describe continuity of care as consisting of

> . . . three essential aspects . . . Firstly it requires a stable care environment, secondly good communication to build a responsible doctor–patient relationship and thirdly the goal of achieving an improvement of the patient's overall health.[110]

Based on the previous discussions, Table 13.2 describes the characteristics of the system dimensions of continuity of care, and Figure 13.4 translates these into a basic systems model, visualising the interconnectedness of the multiple dimensions of continuity – care occurs in the context of the community and its rights and regulations, is influenced by the individual characteristics of the doctor and the patient, both of which shape consultations and their outcomes. The latter, through feedback to the other dimensions modulates and reshapes the continuity of care system.[111]

A complexity approach to continuity deems redundant the question 'Is continuity of care a process or an outcome?'[85] – continuity of care is both.[111] A stable doctor–patient relationship is a *sine qua non*, though it does not necessarily guarantee good health outcomes.[85]

THE INTERCONNECTED NATURE OF CONTINUITY OF CARE

Filling the basic model of continuity of care as illustrated in Figure 13.4 with its agents and constructing a more detailed multiple cause/sign graph diagram helps firstly to visualise the many interconnections between agents and secondly to understand potential interactions between them.

The examples presented in Figures 13.5 and 13.6 are drawn from two different studies, one highlighting the significant interrelationships between high doctor–patient stability and other agents of the continuity system from Hjortdahl's work,[112] the second those agents of the system that are associated with poor doctor–patient stability from Sweeney and Gray's work.[113]

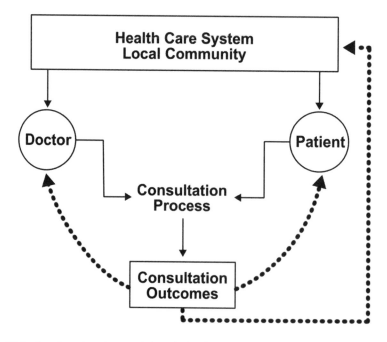

Figure 13.4   A systems-based concept of continuity of care.

TABLE 13.2 The dimensions and system agents of continuity of care

DIMENSION	SYSTEM AGENT
Context of care, including demographics	Healthcare policy
	Healthcare financing
	Doctor–patient ratio
	Accessibility of practice/doctor (rural/urban)
	Socio-economics of the local area
	Access to other healthcare providers
	Time of care, e.g. in-hours surgery versus emergency care
Patient	Attitudes and expectations
	Beliefs
	Prior experiences
	Morbidity
	Self-perceived health
	Cost expectations
Doctor	Attitudes and expectations
	Beliefs
	Prior experiences
	Income expectations
	Knowing the patient
Doctor–patient interaction	Stability of practice
	Stability of relationship
	Consultation length
	Consultation difficulty
	Communication
	Reaching understanding
	Ordering investigations
	Prescribing
	Referring to other providers
Outcomes of care	Ability to cope with illness
	Co-ordination of care
	Appropriateness of care
	Functional health status
	Concordance with treatment plans
	Resource use
	Satisfaction

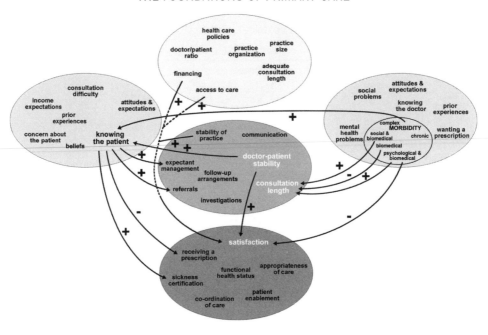

Figure 13.5 Factors associated with good doctor–patient stability. Note: a change in the variable at the beginning of the arrow leads to a change in the same direction '+'/opposite direction '–' of the variable at the end of the arrow.

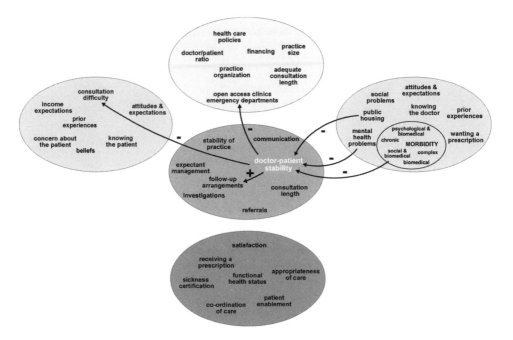

Figure 13.6 Factors associated with poor doctor–patient stability. Note: a change in the variable at the beginning of the arrow leads to a change in the same direction '+'/opposite direction '–' of the variable at the end of the arrow.

UTILITY OF CONTINUITY OF CARE

As Gonella and Herman stated, medical care must lead to improved patient health outcomes.[107] So far no studies have been conducted to demonstrate the improved health outcomes in a continuity environment directly;[85] however, a large number of studies have been conducted using proxy indicators to show these outcomes.

The following tables (Tables 13.3–13.5) detail the findings from Saultz and Lochner's review of the outcomes literature on continuity of care.[114] The tables list only those studies that were evaluated as being of the highest methodological quality (i.e. a score of ≥7 out of 10). Overwhelmingly studies showed an improvement in healthcare processes – more trust in the doctor–patient relationship, more complete documentation of care in the record, improved timing and more indicated preventive care – and outcomes – better compliance with antibiotics, less emergency hospitalisation, decreased rate and length of hospitalisation, fewer days in the intensive care unit (ICU), and improved maternal care with lower neonatal morbidity, better Apgar scores and higher birth weight.

Only diabetes-specific care showed a mixed picture between the personal provider continuity and discontinuity groups; one study showed an improvement in overall care and a reduction in the number having very poor control, though on average there was no difference in glycaemic control; one study showed no difference in overall glycaemic, blood pressure and lipid control; and one study (Table 13.3) showed an inverse relationship between glycaemic control and quality of life.

TABLE 13.3 The dimensions and system agents of continuity of care

OUTCOME MEASURE	EFFECT OF PERSONAL PROVIDER CONTINUITY ON OUTCOME			NO OF STUDIES	STUDY TYPE
	BETTER	NO DIFFERENCE	WORSE	N = 18	
Trust in doctor–patient relationship	Better			1	Correlation
Record documentation	Better			2	Correlation
Preventive care	Influenza vaccination	Mammography, obesity, tobacco use		1	Retrospective
	All preventive issues			2	Correlation
	Pap smear, mammogram, and breast examination			1	Correlation
Compliance with antibiotics	Pharyngitis	Otitis media		1	Prospective
	All conditions			1	Correlation
Emergency hospitalisation	Less			1	Trial
Hospitalisation rate	Decreased, highest continuity – lowest rate			4	Retrospective
ICU days	Fewer			1	Trial

TABLE 13.3 *cont*

OUTCOME MEASURE	EFFECT OF PERSONAL PROVIDER CONTINUITY ON OUTCOME			NO OF STUDIES	STUDY TYPE
	BETTER	NO DIFFERENCE	WORSE	*N* = 18	
Length of hospital stay	Shorter			1	Trial
Neonatal morbidity	More visits and better birth outcomes			1	Retrospective
Apgar score	Better			1	Retrospective
Birth weight	Higher			1	Retrospective
Timeliness of childhood immunisations	Better up to age 15 months			2	Retrospective
Diabetes care	Higher quality of life, but poorer control	HbA_{1c}, lipids, blood pressure complications	Poorer control, but higher quality of life	2	Correlation
	More recommended care, fewer with HbA_{1c} >10%	Average HbA_{1c}		1	Retrospective

TABLE 13.4 The dimensions and system agents of continuity of care

OUTCOME MEASURE	EFFECT OF COMPREHENSIVE CLINIC SETTING ON OUTCOME			NO OF STUDIES	STUDY TYPE
	BETTER	NO DIFFERENCE	WORSE	*N* = 5	
Preventive health visits	Higher			1	Correlation
Preventive health	Pap smears, mammography, breast examination	Well-child visits, blood pressure check in women		1	Correlation
Vaccinations	Only polio was higher			1	Trial
Health behaviours	Lower substance abuse, lower smoking rate	Obesity		1	Correlation
Compliance with antibiotics		No difference		1	Trial
Hospitalisation rate		Higher in comprehensive group in first 6 months, higher in control group after 6 months		1	Trial
Well-child visits	Higher			1	Trial
Illness visits of children	Higher			1	Trial
Functional health		Unchanged in nursing home patients at time of hospitalisation		1	Prospective cohort

A set of five studies compared the outcomes of comprehensive care that did not measure personal provider continuity. The outcomes of this form of care provision were somewhat better in preventive care, but showed no difference in all other outcome measures (*see* Table 13.4). This finding is particularly important as it highlights the substantial benefit associated with the additional quality of personal provider care over and above that associated with a more 'user-friendly' care environment.

Twelve studies examined the cost implications associated with personal provider continuity and all found a significant reduction in overall and specific cost as well as a reduction in resource use (*see* Table 13.5).

Little is known about patients who prefer discontinuity of care. However these studies have shown that patients without a personal provider are a vulnerable group. They are usually younger, less health conscious and less healthy, and seek care for their perceived needs from open access or specialist clinics.[113,115]

TABLE 13.5 The dimensions and system agents of continuity of care

COST MEASURE	EFFECT OF PERSONAL PROVIDER CONTINUITY ON COST			NO OF STUDIES	STUDY TYPE
	LOWER	NO DIFFERENCE	HIGHER	N = 12	
Difficult visits			With low continuity	1	Case–control
Illness visits	With higher continuity			1	Trial
Failure to attend	With higher continuity		With low continuity	1	Case–control
Outpatient services	Fewer ECGs and chest X-rays			3	Trial
	Fewer laboratory tests			1	Trial
	Fewer visits			2	Prospective
	Fewer prescriptions				
Emergency department visits	With higher continuity		With low continuity	2	Retrospective
	With higher continuity			1	Trial
Hospitalisation rate	With higher continuity			4	Retrospective
	With higher continuity			2	Trial
	With higher continuity			1	Prospective
Emergency hospitalisation	With higher continuity			1	Trial
	With higher continuity			1	Correlation
	With higher continuity			1	Case–control
ICU days	With higher continuity			1	Trial
Surgical procedures			With higher continuity	1	Trial
Overall care costs	With higher continuity			2	Retrospective
	With higher continuity			1	Prospective
Drug costs	With higher continuity			1	Trial

SUMMARY POINTS

- General practice/family medicine defines itself by its commitment to the person.
- The person is more important than his disease.
- Illness occurs in the whole context of the person, and conversely affects that whole context.
- The knowledge domains of general practice/family medicine encompass known, knowable, complex and chaos dimensions.
- The personal relationship with and commitment to the patient is the essential building block of general practice/family medicine.
- Patient-centred medicine involves the patient as a partner in the therapeutic relationship and strengthens the patient's self-healing properties.
- Without trust there is no healing relationship.
- Phronesis is gained by experience and reflection, and cannot be condensed to protocols and guidelines.
- Without time there is no healing relationship.
- An important role of the general practitioner/family physician is the advocacy and protection of the patient in the face of 'medical exploitation'.
- Continuity of care is simultaneously a process and an outcome.
- A meaningful therapeutic relationship cannot develop without doctor–patient stability.
- Patients who have a personal doctor achieve better health and better health outcomes.
- Patients who have a personal doctor consume fewer of the scarce healthcare resources.

CHAPTER 14

Emerging patterns

The time has come to give to the study of the responses that the living organism makes to its environment the same dignity and support which is being given at present to the science of parts and reactions isolated from the organism ... Physicians have the overwhelming advantage that bedside experience gives them an awareness of the fundamental needs and potentialities of the human condition ... Medicine has the opportunity to ... [develop] a science of man ... [to] complement the reductionist analysis of structures and mechanisms.

Rene Dubos[116]

Healing is the ultimate purpose of medical care, and thus *shapes the core values* of the medical profession. These values need to be translated into health service policy as well as health service delivery to create an effective and efficient health service. At a time of competing, and at times diabolically opposed, interests in society, different convictions interfere with the core principles of medical care.

Four main patterns emerge from the discussions in this section on healing. The first is a crisis of confidence in one's health. Ninety per cent of the community experiences illness in any given month, and more than one-third of these seek medical care. The epidemic in illness though contradicts the steady prevalence of serious disease requiring specialist health services.

A second pattern reflects the discomfort with the life experiences across the continuum of health–illness–disease and death. In the traditional Cartesian reductionist paradigm all deviations from perfect wellbeing tend to promote the creation of new (objective) diseases combined with their (scientific and technological) therapies. Conceptualising health and illness as a personal balanced state within a somato-psycho-socio-semiotic framework shifts the focus back onto the traditional notions of health, health care and healing.

Care and healing are based on the powers of a *personal relationship*, the third pattern,

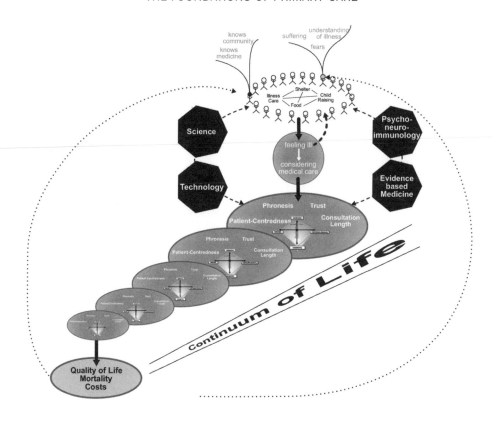

Figure 14.1 Personal health and personalised health care in the context of divergent societal demands.

between doctor and patient which are better measurable by qualitative indicators such as quality of life measures; nevertheless these descriptive qualities have their biomedical correlates in psychoneuroimmunological parameters. In many Western societies, technology and excessive regulation of medical care interfere with the healing function of medicine.

The fourth pattern describes the processes of *continuing* and *person-centred care*. These are the foundations of trust and security in the therapeutic relationship, as much as they are the basis for wise decision making in the context of the individual patient. Person-centred continuing care is no more time-consuming than episodic and fragmented care, but besides of being more effective it is less resource intensive.

These four patterns co-exist and shape the healthcare system. What is needed is *reaffirmation of the core values in health care*. Core values shape complex adaptive systems, and thus allow a healthcare system to emerge that can successfully deal with divergent views and demands. This theme will be further explored in Section 5 of this book. Figure 14.1 illustrates that the fundamental needs in society for health care remain unchanged as does the need for personalised health care. What has changed are secondary concerns that impeach on the proper functioning of the healing process.

FURTHER READING

Balint M. *The Doctor, His Patient and the Illness.* Edinburgh, London, Melbourne and New York: Churchill Livingstone, 1957.

Feinstein AR. *Clinical Judgement.* New York: The Williams & Wilkins Company, 1967.

McWhinney IR. *A Textbook of Family Medicine.* New York, Oxford: Oxford University Press, 1989.

Stewart M, Brown JB, Weston WW *et al. Patient-centered Medicine.* Thousand Oaks: Sage Publications, 1995.

REFERENCES

1 Causes of Death 2003: Australian Bureau of Statistics. www.abs.gov.au/Ausstats/abs@.nsf/0/2093da6935db138fca2568a9001393c9?OpenDocument (accessed 3 July 2006).

2 Causes of Death 2000: Fiji Islands Bureau of Statistics. www.statsfiji.gov.fj/Social/health_cdeath.htm (accessed 3 July 2006).

3 White K, Williams F and Greenberg B. The ecology of medical care. *New England Journal of Medicine.* 1961; **265**: 885–92.

4 Green L, Fryer G, Yawn B, Lanier D and Dovey S. The ecology of medical care revisited. *New England Journal of Medicine.* 2001; **344**: 2021–5.

5 Turnberg L. Science, society and the perplexed physician. *Journal of the Royal College of Physicians of London* 2000; **34**: 569–75.

6 Fugelli P. Clinical practice: between Aristotle and Cochrane. *Schweizerische Medizinische Wochenschrift.* 1998; **128**: 184–8.

7 Pellegrino E and Thomasma D. *A Philosophical Basis of Medical Practice. Towards a Philosophy and Ethic of the Healing Professions.* New York Oxford: Oxford University Press, 1981.

8 Rosenberg C. Disease in history: frames and framers. *Milbank Quarterly.* 1989; **67**(Suppl 1): 1–15.

9 Rosenberg C. The tyranny of diagnosis: specific entities and individual experience. *Milbank Quarterly.* 2002; **80**: 237–60.

10 Mackenbach JP. Carl von Linne, Thomas McKeown, and the inadequacy of disease classifications. *European Journal of Public Health.* 2004; **14**: 225.

11 Croockshank F. The theory of diagnosis. Part I. *Lancet.* 1926; **November 6**: 939–42.

12 Fisher E and Welch H. Avoiding the unintended consequences of growth in medical care. How might more be worse? *Journal of the American Medical Association.* 1999; **281**: 446–53.

13 Schwartz L and Woloshin S. Changing disease definitions: implications for disease prevalence. *Effective Clinical Practice.* 1999; **2**: 76–85.

14 PLoS Medicine. Disease Mongering. *PLoS Medicine.* 2006; **3**: http://collections.plos.org/diseasemongering-2006.php (accessed 4 July 2006).

15 Westin S and Heath I. Thresholds for normal blood pressure and serum cholesterol. *British Medical Journal.* 2005; **330**: 1461–2.

16 Getz L, Kirkengen A, Hetlevik I, Romundstad S and Sigurdsson J. Ethical dilemmas arising from implementation of the European guidelines on cardiovascular disease prevention in clinical practice. A descriptive epidemiological study. *Scandinavian Journal of Primary Health Care.* 2004; **22**: 2002–8.

17 Baron R. An introduction to medical phenomenology: I can't hear you while I'm listening. *Annals of Internal Medicine.* 1985; **103**: 606–11.

18 Meador C. The art and science of nondisease. *New England Journal of Medicine.* 1965; **272**: 92–5.

19 Mayou R and Sharpe M. Treating medically unexplained physical symptoms. *British Medical Journal.* 1997; **315**: 561–2.

20 McWhinney I. Family medicine in perspective. *New England Journal of Medicine.* 1975; **293**: 176–81.

21 Mead N and Bower P. Patient-centredness: a conceptual framework and review of the empirical literature. *Social Science and Medicine.* 2000; **51**: 1087–110.

22 Lekander M, Elofsson S, Neve I-M, Hansson L-O and Unden A-L. Self-rated health is related to levels of circulating cytokines. *Psychosomatic Medicine.* 2004; **66**: 559–63.

23 Kiecolt-Glaser J and Glaser R. Psychoneuroimmunology and health consequences: data and shared mechanisms. *Psychosomatic Medicine.* 1995; **57**: 269–74.

24 McWhinney I. The importance of being different. William Pickles Lecture 1996. *British Journal of General Practice.* 1996; **46**: 433–6.

25 Taylor R. *Medicine out of Control.* Melbourne: Sun Books, 1979.

26 World Health Organization. Declaration of Alma-Ata. International Conference on Primary Health Care, Alma-Ata, USSR, 6–12 September 1978. Geneva: World Health Organization, 1978.

27 Bentzen N. WONCA international glossary for general practice/family medicine. *Family Practice.* 1995; **12**: 341–69.

28 Illich I. *Limits to Medicine. Medical nemesis: the expropriation of health.* London: Marion Boyars Book, 1976.

29 Engel G. The clinical application of the biopsychosocial model. *American Journal of Psychiatry.* 1980; **137**: 535–44.

30 Uexküll TV and Pauli H. The mind-body problem in medicine. *Advances: Journal of the Institute for the Advancement of Health.* 1986; **3**: 158–74.

31 Pauli H, White K and McWhinney I. Medical education, research, and scientific thinking in the 21st century (Part two of three). *Education for Health (Abingdon).* 2000; **13**: 165–72.

32 Sturmberg J. How to teach holistic care – meeting the challenge of complexity in clinical practice. *Education for Health (Abingdon).* 2005; **18**: 236–45.

33 Sturmberg J, Martin C and Moes M. Defining health – a dynamic balance model. Submitted 2006.

34 Toye F, Barlow J, Wright C and Lamb S. Personal meanings in the construction of need for total knee replacement. *Social Science and Medicine.* 2006; **63**: 43–53.

35 Cannon H. Stresses and strains of homeostasis. *American Journal of Medical Science.* 1935; **189**: 1–14.

36 Antonovsky A. The structure and properties of the sense of coherence scale. *Social Science and Medicine.* 1993; **36**: 725–33.

37 Sturmberg J and Piterman L. *The Principles of General Practice.* Melbourne: Department of General Practice, Monash University, 2005.

38 Malterud K. The art and science of clinical knowledge: evidence beyond measures and numbers. *Lancet.* 2001; **358**: 397–400.

39 McCormick J. The contribution of science to medicine. *Perspectives in Biology and Medicine.* 1993; **36**: 315–22.

40 Feinstein A. *Clinical Judgement.* New York: The Williams & Wilkins Company, 1967.

41 Elmore J, Wells C, Lee C, Howard D and Feinstein A. Variability in radiologists' interpretation of mammograms. *New England Journal of Medicine.* 1994; **331**: 1493–9.

42 Gottlieb E. The great x-ray mystery. *JPO: The Journal of Practical Orthodontics.* 1969; **3**: 486–93.

43 Young N, Naryshkin S, Atkinson B *et al.* Interobserver variability of cervical smears with squamous-cell abnormalities: a Philadelphia study. *Diagnostic Cytopathology.* 1994; **11**: 352–7.

44 Cochrane AWMB. *One Man's Medicine.* London: BMJ (Memoir Club), 1989, p. 82.

45 Upshur R. If not evidence, then what? Or does medicine really need a base? *Journal of Evaluation in Clinical Practice.* 2002; **8**: 113–19.

46 Cassel E. *The Healer's Art.* Cambridge, MA: The MIT Press, 1985.

47 McWhinney I. Medical knowledge and the rise of technology. *Journal of Medicine and Philosophy.* 1978; **3**: 293–304.

48 Stephens G. *The Intellectual Basis of Family Practice.* Tucson, Arizona: Winter Publishing Co, 1982.

49 Hart J. Expectations of health care: promoted, managed or shared? *Health Expectations.* 1998; **1**: 3–13.

50 Greenhalgh T and Hurwitz B. Narrative based medicine: why study narrative? *British Medical Journal.* 1999; **318**: 48–50.

51 Solomon G and Moos R. Emotions, immunity, and disease: a speculative theoretical integration. *Archives of General Psychiatry.* 1964; **11**: 657–74.

52 Kiecolt-Glaser J, McGuire L, Robles T and Glaser R. Psychoneuroimmunology: psychological influences on immune function and health. *Journal of Consulting and Clinical Psychology.* 2002; **70**: 537–47.

53 Reiser S. *The Shortcomings of Technology.* Cambridge: Cambridge University Press, 1982.

54 Fredriksen S. Instrumental colonisation in modern medicine. *Medicine, Health Care and Philosophy.* 2003; **6**: 287–96.

55 Guadagnoli E, Hauptman P, Ayanian J *et al.* Variation in the use of cardiac procedures after acute myocardial infarction. *New England Journal of Medicine.* 1995; **333**: 573–8.

56 Feinstein A. Statistical reductionism and clinicians' delinquencies in humanistic research. *Clinical Pharmacology and Therapeutics.* 1999; **66**: 211–17.

57 Polanyi M. *Personal Knowledge. Towards a Post-Critical Philosophy.* London: Routledge, 1958.

58 Daly J and McDonald I. *The Social Impact of Echocardiography.* Canberra: Australian Institute of Health and Welfare, 1993.

59 Hampton J, Harrison M, Mitchell J, Prichard J and Seymour C. Relative contributions of history-taking, physical examination, and laboratory investigation to diagnosis and management of medical outpatients. *British Medical Journal.* 1975; **2**: 486–9.

60 Tonelli M. Integrating evidence into clinical practice: an alternative to evidence-based approaches. *Journal of Evaluation in Clinical Practice.* 2006; **12**: 248–56.

61 Cochrane A. *Effectiveness and Efficiency. Random reflections on health services.* London: The Nuffield Provincial Hospitals Trust, 1972.

62 Worrall J. What evidence in evidence-based medicine. *Philosophy of Science*. 2002; **69**: S316–S330. www.lse.ac.uk/collections/CPNSS/pdf/DP_withCover_Causality/CTR01-02-C.pdf (accessed 4 July 2006).

63 Lau J, Antman E, Jimenez-Silva J *et al.* Cumulative meta-analysis of therapeutic trials for myocardial infarction. *New England Journal of Medicine*. 1992; **327**: 248–54.

64 Pruessner H, Hensel W and Rasco T. The scientific basis of generalist medicine. *Academic Medicine*. 1992; **67**: 232–5.

65 Sackett D, Rosenberg W, Gray J, Haynes R and Richardson W. Evidence based medicine: what it is and what it isn't. *British Medical Journal*. 1996; **312**: 71–2.

66 Evidence-Based Medicine Working Group. Evidence-based medicine. a new approach to teaching the practice of medicine. *Journal of the American Medical Association*. 1992; **268**: 2420–5.

67 Tannenbaum S. What physicians know. *New England Journal of Medicine*. 1993; **329**: 1268–71.

68 Feinstein A and Horwitz R. Problems in the 'evidence' of 'evidence-based medicine'. *American Journal of Medicine*. 1997; **103**: 529–35.

69 Naylor C. Grey zones of clinical practice: some limits to evidence-based medicine. *Lancet*. 1995; **345**: 840–2.

70 Britton A, McKee M, Black N *et al.* Threats to applicability of randomised trials: exclusions and selective participation. *Journal of Health Services Research and Policy*. 1999; **4**: 112–21.

71 Lauritzen T, Mainz J and Lassen J. From science to everyday clinical practice. Need for systematic evaluation of research findings. *Scandinavian Journal of Primary Health Care*. 1999; **17**: 6–10.

72 Concato J, Shah N and Horwitz R. Randomized, controlled trials, observational studies, and the hierarchy of research designs. *New England Journal of Medicine*. 2000; **342**: 1887–92.

73 Bogaty P and Brophy J. Numbers needed to treat (needlessly?). *Lancet*. 2005; **365**: 1307–8.

74 McCormack J and Greenhalgh T. Seeing what you want to see in randomised controlled trials: versions and perversions of UKPDS data. *British Medical Journal*. 2000; **320**: 1720–3.

75 Hjortdahl P. Continuity of care: general practitioners' knowledge about, and sense of responsibility toward their patients. *Family Practice*. 1992; **9**: 3–8.

76 Fugelli P. Trust – in general practice. *British Journal of General Practice*. 2001; **51**: 575–9.

77 Kurtz C and Snowden D. The new dynamics of strategy: sense-making in a complex and complicated world. *IBM Systems Journal*. 2003; **42**: 462–83.

78 Kleinman A. *Patients and Healers in the Context of Cultures*. Los Angeles: University of California Press, 1980.

79 Westin S. The market is a strange creature: family medicine meeting the challenges of the changing political and socioeconomic structure. *Family Practice*. 1995; **12**: 394–401.

80 Stewart M. Effective physician–patient communication and health outcomes: a review. *Canadian Medical Association Journal*. 1995; **152**: 1423–33.

81 Krupat E, Bell R, Kravitz R, Thom D and Azari R. When physicians and patients think alike: patient-centered beliefs and their impact on satisfaction and trust. *Journal of Family Practice*. 2001; **50**: 1057–62.

82 Chenail R, Douthit P, Gale J *et al.* 'It's probably nothing serious, but . . .': parents' interpretation of referral to pediatric cardiologists. *Health Communication.* 1990; **2**: 165–88.

83 Kaplan S, Greenfield S and Ware J. Assessing the effects of physician-patient interactions on the outcomes of chronic disease. *Medical Care.* 1989; **27**(Suppl): S110–S127.

84 Roter D, Stewart M, Putman S *et al.* Communication patterns of primary care physicians. *Canadian Medical Association Journal.* 1997; **277**: 350–6.

85 Christakis DA. Continuity of care: process or outcome? *Annals of Family Medicine.* 2003; **1**: 131–3.

86 von Bultzingslowen I, Eliasson G, Sarvimaki A, Mattsson B and Hjortdahl P. Patients' views on interpersonal continuity in primary care: a sense of security based on four core foundations. *Family Practice.* 2006; **23**: 210–19.

87 Beckman H and Frankel R. The effect of physician behavior on the collection of data. *Annals of Internal Medicine.* 1984; **101**: 692–6.

88 Safran D, Taira D, Rogers W *et al.* Linking primary care performance to outcomes of care. *Family Practice.* 1998; **47**: 213–20.

89 Schers H, van den Hoogen H, Bor H, Grol R and van den Bosch W. Familiarity with a GP and patients' evaluations of care. A cross-sectional study. *Family Practice.* 2005; **22**: 15–19.

90 Bonds D, Camacho F, Bell R *et al.* The association of patient trust and self-care among patients with diabetes mellitus. *BMC Family Practice.* 2004; **5**(26).

91 Ewig S. Was ist ein guter Arzt? *Frankfurter Allgemeine Sonntagszeitung.* 2006; **7 May**: 73–4.

92 Lin C-T, Albertson G, Schilling L *et al.* Is patients' perception of time spent with the physician a determinant of ambulatory patient satisfaction? *Annals of Internal Medicine.* 2001; **161**: 1437–42.

93 Howie J, Heaney D, Maxwell M *et al.* Quality at general practice consultations: cross sectional survey. *British Medical Journal.* 1999; **319**: 738–43.

94 Blumenthal D, Causino N, Chang Y *et al.* The duration of ambulatory visits to physicians. *Journal of Family Practice.* 1999; **48**: 264–71.

95 Wilson A and Childs S. The relationship between consultation length, process and outcomes in general practice: a systematic review. *British Journal of General Practice.* 2002; **52**: 1012–20.

96 Freeman G, Horder J, Howie J *et al.* Evolving general practice consultation in Britain: issues of length and context. *British Medical Journal.* 2002; **324**: 820–2.

97 Gulbrandsen P, Fugelli P, Sandvik L and Hjortdahl P. Influence of social problems on management in general practice: multipractice questionnaire survey. *British Medical Journal.* 1998; **317**: 28–32.

98 Hennen B. Continuity of care in family practice. Part 1: Dimensions of continuity. *Journal of Family Practice.* 1975; **2**: 371–2.

99 McWhinney I. Continuity of care in family practice. Part 2: Implications of continuity. *Journal of Family Practice.* 1975; **2**: 373–4.

100 Hansen M. Continuity of care in family practice. Part 3: Measurement and evaluation of continuity of care. *Journal of Family Practice.* 1975; **2**: 439–44.

101 Geyman J. Continuity of care in family practice. Part 4: Implementing continuity in a family practice residency program. *Journal of Family Practice.* 1975; **2**: 445–7.

102 Rogers J and Curtis P. The concept and measurement of continuity in primary care. *American Journal of Public Health*. 1980; **70**: 122–7.

103 Becker M, Drachman R and Kirscht J. A field experiement to evaluate various outcomes of continuity of physician care. *American Journal of Public Health*. 1974; **64**: 1062–70.

104 Hjortdahl P. Ideology and reality of continuity of care. *Family Medicine*. 1990; **22**: 361–4.

105 Banahan B and Banahan BI. Continuity as an attitudianal contract. *Journal of Family Practice*. 1981; **12**: 767–8.

106 McWhinney I. *A Textbook of Family Medicine*. New York Oxford: Oxford University Press, 1989.

107 Gonnella J and Herman M. Continuity of care. *Journal of the American Medical Association*. 1980; **243**: 352–4.

108 Haggerty J, Reid R, Freeman G *et al*. Continuity of care: a multidisciplinary review. *British Medical Journal*. 2003; **327**: 1219–21.

109 Saultz J. Defining and measuring interpersonal continuity of care. *Annals of Family Medicine*. 2003; **1**: 134–43.

110 Sturmberg J. Continuity of care: towards a definition based on experiences of practising GPs. *Family Practice*. 2000; **17**: 16–20.

111 Sturmberg J. Continuity of care: a systems-based approach. *Asia Pacific Family Medicine*. 2003; **2**: 136–42.

112 Hjortdahl P. *Continuity of Care in General Practice. A study related to ideology and reality of continuity of care in Norwegian general practice*. Oslo: University of Oslo, 1992.

113 Sweeney K and Gray D. Patients who do not receive continuity of care from their general practitioner – are they a vulnerable group? *British Journal of General Practice*. 1995; **45**: 133–5.

114 Saultz JW and Lochner J. Interpersonal continuity of care and care outcomes: a critical review. *Annals of Family Medicine*. 2005; **3**: 159–66.

115 Devroey D, Coigniez P, Vandevoorde J, Kartounian J and Betz W. Prevention and follow-up of cardiovascular disease among patients without a personal GP. *Family Practice*. 2003; **20**: 420–4.

116 Dubos R. *Man Adapting*. New Haven, CT: Yale, 1965.

History	Philosophy	The Practice of Medicine	Social	Primary Care
Social Construct of Health Public Health Infrastructure	Husserl	Personal Relationship Phronesis Continuity of Care Care Co-ordination Quality of Life	Social Capital	Common Goal Integrated BUT Diverse Solutions
Shaman/Medicine Man Hippocrates of Cos Care for the Whole Patient	Pellegrino		Income Inequality	
Broad Education Apprenticeship Model of Learning	Cynefin Knowledge Model	SOMATIC SOCIAL PSYCHOLOGICAL SEMIOTIC	Employment	
Knowledge of Disease School of Cnidus	Cartesian Dualism ←→ Complexity Popper	Science & Technology	Access	Personal Health Gain

SECTION FOUR

The social function of medicine: the interdependence of health in society

Medicine is practised in the real world and is deeply embedded in the culture of our societies. The many factors that make up societal life all directly and indirectly impact on our health and illness experiences. Patients bring these experiences into the medical encounter, which in turn impact on the consultation processes and consultation outcomes, and these in turn feed back and shape the expectations and experiences of communities.

There are many different societal factors that impact on the *health* of individuals and communities, not all of which can be explored in this book. The topics alluded to are necessarily selective and solely aim to illustrate some of the additional complexities faced by community-based doctors. The issues discussed are those that have a well-recognised impact on health even though their mechanisms (in a reductionist way) are not fully understood, and may well only be accessible within a complex adaptive systems framework.

Societal issues are clearly *value laden*. Readers will need to consider this reality in the context of their own society. Are societal values *clearly articulated* by political and medical leaders? Are leaders *acting in accordance with the values of society*? Is there a need

147

to engage in *discourse with one's patients* when confronted with health problems that are a consequence of social issues?

The first chapter in this section, using HIV/AIDS as an example, illustrates how a disease shapes society, and how societies shape a disease. Inevitably HIV/AIDS also demonstrates the importance of (or lack of) social capital and other community resources in being able to cope with disease on an individual and community level.

The next chapter asks the difficult question 'Do doctors have an obligation to speak out against social and socio-economic disadvantage?'. A number of examples illustrate the consequences of socio-economic disadvantage on the lifelong health of people.

The effects of 'the market' on health care are explored in the following chapter, alluding to another equally difficult question 'How should health care be financed, and what is the impact of the choice on the health and economy of a community?'. The intrusion of 'the market' into health care has – completely inappropriately – increased the level of anxiety about health and dying in the community, resulting in many unnecessary treatments and associated iatrogenic morbidity and mortality.

The final chapter in this section focuses on income inequality as a specific factor of social disadvantage. Relative income inequality has a more pronounced effect on health than absolute income levels, and a small reduction in community-based income inequality would achieve a substantial improvement in age-adjusted all-cause mortality.

CHAPTER 15

The social nature of health and medicine

The very beginnings of medicine have been social in origin; medical care was constructed as a means of strengthening the survival chances of one's nuclear group. The need to explore medicine, and particularly the disease notion, as a social construct is highlighted by Charles Rosenberg:

> There has never been a time that humankind has not suffered from sickness, and the physician's specialized social role has developed in response to it . . . every aspect of an individual's social identity is constructed – and thus also is disease.[1]

. . . and for that matter health. Earlier it has been shown how easily the line between health and disease can be altered, and how much these changes impact on individual and community wellbeing, affordability of sickness care and health economics, especially in market-oriented health systems, and how redefinition of disease impacts on social and health service policy.[1,2]

The interconnectedness of these diverse *mental mindsets* has an additional historical and political dimension. Not only have certain diseases been marginalised in terms of knowledge generation,[1] but also economic self-interests of large corporations restricted certain medical treatments, like anti-retrovirals or antimalarials, being available to marginalised communities.

SOCIAL RESPONSES TO DISEASE

Not only are diseases shaped by society, diseases shape society. The complex interactions between health and disease are further reflected in the complex interactions between disease and society.

The approach to tuberculosis in the late 19th and early 20th centuries shows the social adaptation to the most common health problem of that time. Health authorities required isolation, but not all doctors agreed with this approach. Institutions struggled to find frameworks to accommodate tuberculosis into their endeavours. The medical profession equally struggled; while the early diagnosis posed a challenge, those with established and advanced disease were seen as unrewarding patients – they didn't get better. Patients on the other hand had a slow decline and struggled on to maintain as normal a life as possible driven by the need to support their families. Treatment options were few and the sanatorium the only promise for remission, but patients ordinarily were not keen to be admitted until their needs and that of their then exhausted families couldn't be met in any other way.[1]

Social response to disease occurs on two levels, one demanding changes of the individual, the other demanding changes by the state. An example for the former relates to sexuality and sexually transmissible infections *requiring change to individual health behaviour* – varying from safe sex education to demanding sexual abstinence; an example for the latter relates to water-borne diseases like typhoid or cholera *requiring public agency responses* – microbiological surveillance, repair or construction of water and sanitation infrastructure, vaccination programmes and so forth.[1]

DISEASE SHAPING SOCIAL RESPONSES

Disease itself can become a trigger for complex changes in social attitude and behaviour for patients, doctors and society at large. The classical example, leprosy, even today means that the affected will experience rejection and isolation from society.

In many Western societies, our dealings with people who have alcohol and drug problems, or who are affected by mental illness, are other examples of social stigma as well as social neglect.

HIV/AIDS has created major challenges to the social fabric of many countries. The opening speeches to the 13th, 14th and 15th International AIDS conferences illustrate the complex interactions between societal views on the disease and the influence on shaping particular social responses.

Thabo Mbeki, South Africa's president, in his opening address in 2000 pointed to extreme poverty as the main driver for HIV/AIDS:[3]

> Let me tell you a storyt that the World Health Organization told the world in 1995. I will tell this story in the words used by the World Health Organization.
>
> This is the story: 'The world's biggest killer and the greatest cause of ill-health and suffering across the globe is listed almost at the end of the International Classification of Diseases. It is given the code Z59.5 – extreme poverty . . . HIV and AIDS are having a devastating effect on young people.
>
> In many countries in the developing world, up to two-thirds of all new infections are among people aged 15–24. Overall it is estimated that half the global HIV infections have been in people under 25 years with 60% of infections of females occurring by the age

of 20. Thus the hopes and lives of a generation, the breadwinners, providers and parents of the future, are in jeopardy.

. . . One of the consequences of this crisis is the deeply disturbing phenomenon of the collapse of immune systems among millions of our people, such that their bodies have no natural defence against attack by many viruses and bacteria.

Clearly, if we, as African countries, had the level of development to enable us to gather accurate statistics about our own countries, our morbidity and mortality figures would tell a story that would truly be too frightening to contemplate.

As I listened and heard the whole story told about our own country, it seemed to me that we could not blame everything on a single virus.

. . . We look forward to the results of this important work, which will help us to ensure that we achieve better results in terms of saving the lives of our people and improving the lives of millions. In the meantime, we will continue to intensify our own campaign against AIDS, including: a sustained public awareness campaign encouraging safe sex and the use of condoms; a better focused programme targeted at the reduction and elimination of poverty and the improvement of the nutritional standards of our people; a concerted fight against the so-called opportunistic diseases, including TB and all sexually transmitted diseases; a humane response to people living with HIV and AIDS as well as the orphans in our society; contributing to the international effort to develop an AIDS vaccine; and, further research on anti-retroviral drugs.

. . . The world's biggest killer and the greatest cause of ill health and suffering across the globe, including South Africa, is extreme poverty.[3]

Dr Jordi Casabona, Director of the AIDS Epidemiology Study Center of the Department of Health of Catalonia in his 2002 opening remarks pointed to the need to integrate the various aspects of addressing the AIDS epidemic through policy initiatives:[4]

For the past 21 years we have been exponentially gaining more information on the HIV virus and its determinants for spread, including, of course, the social-economic ones. Nevertheless, we know that all this information and knowledge is useless if it is not translated into effective progress . . . I am also convinced there is more knowledge and global political will than ever, and that we have a unique historical opportunity to translate them into economic commitments and scientific-based action.

. . . We encourage you to share and discuss the social-economical and political barriers to prevention, treatment, and care access, and the approaches to overcome them. Our discussions together will eventually help in sustaining and scaling-up effective responses to AIDS. Therefore, we also welcome the presence of so many political leaders that we will have with us this week. Because we believe that effective action cannot happen without science, not without activism or policy, we have put together bridging sessions that will cover special relevant topics in an original, integrated approach, from basic science to policy.[4]

Thaksin Shinawatra, Thailand's Prime Minister, based his 2004 opening remarks on his personal experiences with HIV/AIDS patients.[5] He emphasised the need for prevention, especially the strategy of free distribution of anti-retrovirals to all HIV-infected individuals, but also highlighted the need for society to accept and reintegrate the diseased back into their communities and workplaces:

> Based on the evidence witnessed with my own eyes and reinforced by close personal contact, I would like to declare, here and now – in front of you all – that I will never cease my commitment to support universal coverage of Anti-Retroviral [ARV] treatment to people with HIV and AIDS. It is the very least we can do.
>
> . . . I would therefore like to urge all governments around the world to do their utmost to provide ARV treatment to those who need them. We are in an emergency situation. Without ARV, some 8000 people will die from AIDS every day. Some may be our friends, our neighbors, or even someone we love. But with ARV, we can immediately put a stop to this dismal problem.
>
> . . . Let me add that, I am now thinking beyond the ARV program. When people with HIV and AIDS have been brought back to their healthy lives, this is not the end of the story. They also need to go back to work, and to re-enter the mainstream of society. Therefore, my Government has created a new program aimed at vocational training and supporting them with jobs to earn income for their families. This program should be along the same lines as the ARV program.
>
> However, whether this program will work or not depends also on the acceptance of the general public towards people with HIV and AIDS. I would therefore like to call on all the people in Thailand and throughout the world to give a chance to people with HIV and AIDS. Give them an opportunity to live and work and lead a normal life in their communities, as they are truly one of the members of our society, just like you and me.
>
> . . . There is no time for complacency; no time to rest on our laurels. It would be a crime to let HIV continue to spread, while we already know how to interrupt it. It would be an even greater crime to let people suffer from AIDS, without any access to treatment, while effective medicine is readily available. We cannot ignore the reality that there are still large numbers of people with no access to information and prevention products.[5]

These responses highlight how complex issues are broken down into seemingly simple and straightforward ones. One has to acknowledge that each of the speakers highlighted valid aspects in handling the HIV epidemic, but one must also stress that all of these issues are interacting with each other, and that no single response alone is going to achieve the desired result. In fact focusing all energy on one issue alone may achieve either nothing or even may make the situation worse.

Framing of the problem, i.e. how to ask questions about the problem, shapes the solutions; Figure 15.1 and Table 15.1 provides an example of the difference between a simple and a complex approach to HIV. Brazil saw HIV as a complex problem and responded accordingly, and by 2000 achieved an infection rate of 0.6%, whereas many other comparable countries have infection rates of up to 25%.[6]

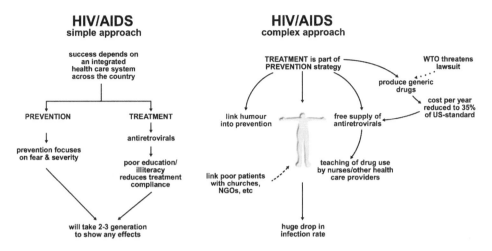

Figure 15.1   Simple and complex approaches to HIV/AIDS in developing countries

CONSTRUCTING HEALTH AND DISEASE IN THE CONSULTATION

On a microlevel, Daly and McDonald showed how the interaction between doctor and patient in the consultation lead to different constructions of health and disease in patients referred for an echocardiographic evaluation of their heart.[7] Patients' anxieties were partly resolved by the reassurance of their heart being normal; however, the reassurance in the majority did not lead to a full understanding or elimination of their perceived problem. On the other hand doctors (cardiologists) firmly believed that having provided *technical* evidence of a normal heart should readily be able to *fix* the patients' concerns. To explore the meaning behind the patient's concern was viewed as either irrelevant or inappropriate, highlighting their *linear scientific* construct rather than the patient's *complex social and individual* construct of health. To integrate the new information into the *complex system of personal health* is most effectively achieved through a narrative approach; communication is the tool to establish the connections with the other agents in the system that ultimately leads to a new understanding of health (*see* Table 15.1).[8]

TABLE 15.1 Comparing the simple and complex approach to HIV (adapted from Glouberman and Zimmerman[6])

SIMPLE APPROACH	COMPLEX APPROACH
Q: With our limited resources, should we focus more on prevention or treatment? Or what are the resources for an effective prevention/ treatment programme?	Q: How can we achieve our prevention goals while treating all of those currently infected?
A: With our limited resources, we should focus more on prevention than treatment.	A: We will find a way to provide treatment to all who need it by dramatically reducing costs.
A: We cannot provide treatment to all when the costs are so high. Choices must be made.	A: Prevention will be part of treatment and treatment will allow us 'access' to the population for prevention strategies.

TECHNOLOGY REPLACING COMMUNICATION

Stethoscopes, X-rays and electrocardiograms have transcended human senses. Technology has enabled doctors *to see* disease in the living, and *to use* it to enable cure; technology has *transformed* our *social understanding* of health and disease.

The assimilation of *sense-transcending technologies* has intruded into our lifeworld. This self-transcending nature has made us no longer trust our own senses. Technology speaks for itself and has replaced the need for interpersonal communication. Fredricksen called this transcending nature of technology the colonisation of the lifeworld:

> Medical technology causes colonisation because it is embedded in a context that changes the way we think and act; a context that makes it possible for a person to understand that he now has become a patient. And the actual impact of medicine has been even more profound. Modern medicine has turned us all into 'proto-patients'. Without further ado, we accept that we can become patients any minute, even if we do not experience any symptoms at all.[9]

The consequences of these developments in society are reflected in the increasing number of people feeling ill and being concerned about their health, even though the incidence of serious disease has not change at all.[10,11] Besides the impact on the personal enjoyment of life, medicalisation of all life experiences places an insurmountable burden on the limited economic resources available within society.[1]

SOCIAL CAPITAL

Social capital is created from the myriad of everyday interactions between people. Social capital is not owned by any organisation, the market or the state; however, all of them can engage in its production.[12] Despite its implied economic notion,[13] social capital is defined in several non-economic ways:

- A set of 'horizontal associations' between people, social networks, networks of civic engagement and associated norms of reciprocity.[14]
- A variety of entities that have two elements in common, they consist of some

aspect of social structure, and they facilitate certain actions; this definition entails a 'vertical association'.[15]

- The social and political environment that allows norms to develop, and that shapes the social structure. This view embraces the informal nature of the above definitions and extends them by including formal structures like government, political regimes, the rule of law, the court system, civil and political liberties.[16,17]

Grootaert highlights that social capital can only be acquired by a group of people and requires co-operation amongst them.[13] He describes the implications of this as follows:

> This gives social capital an inevitable public good character and has implications for its production. In particular, like all public goods, it will tend to be underproduced relative to the social optimum unless the group responsible for its production can internalize the externality involved. This is why horizontal associations, characterized by equitable power sharing among members, tend to be more successful at generating social capital. Members are more likely to contribute because they have a better chance of obtaining their fair share of the benefit.[13]

Recently the concept of social capital has been further refined by Szreter and Woolcock, who distinguish between three kinds of social relationship:
- *bonding*: relationships between socially similar groups
- *bridging*: relationships between socially dissimilar groups
- *linking*: relationships between individuals and groups that are explicitly unequal (e.g. local governments and citizenry).[18]

Social capital resources can be described by six social capital indicators: social trust (bonding); trust in public and private institutions (linking); neighbourhood integration (bonding and bridging); neighbourhood alienation (lack of bonding and bridging); neighbourhood safety; and political participation.[19]

SOCIAL CAPITAL AND HEALTH

Disruption of social capital is evidenced by lower interpersonal trust between citizens, and less reciprocity and participation in civic and voluntary associations. A high level of social capital has been associated with greater participation in civic life, the prevention of crime and delinquency, and the maintenance of population health.[20]

Although a link between social capital and health has been established (Table 15.2 provides an example), the mechanisms and the direction are not consistent. While ecological studies have consistently shown a positive association between higher levels of social capital with higher levels of health, findings from multilevel studies (individual health nested within areas that vary in their level of social capital) have found mixed and multidirectional associations with health.[21]

TABLE 15.2 Factors associated with self-rated health (compiled from Poortinga[22])

FAIR/POOR/VERY POOR SELF-RATED HEALTH	VERY GOOD/GOOD SELF-RATED HEALTH
Old age	
Economically inactive people	
Social class gradient	Professional and intermediate
skilled manual	
partly and unskilled manual	
	Owning house
Low level of trust	High level of trust
Low level of civic participation	Medium to high level of civic participation
Some or severe lack of social support	High levels of social support

A surprising finding emerged from a study into self-rated health and area-based social capital in Tasmania/Australia that confirmed the association between socio-economic disadvantage and poor health; however, the association was independent of the local area's social capital, leading the authors to conclude that redistribution of resources (physical infrastructure, public education, tax transfers) to individuals living in disadvantaged areas would be more helpful in improving their health.[19]

Social capital, though not yet precisely defined, adds another dimension to the individual health experience. The health effects appear to be contextual, and the observation of diverse findings in various communities adds to the complexities of understanding the social construct of health. The latter examples in addition would indicate that health improvements for some are not achievable by more medical care but rather by improvements in social infrastructure.

SUMMARY POINTS

- Diseases are shaped by society, and so are societies shaped by their diseases.
- Diseases and their prevention and treatment can only fully be understood within the complexities of society.
- The consultation is the place where patients construct their personal disease and illness understanding.
- Over-reliance on technology infiltrates the experience and the sense-making processes of doctor and patient alike.
- Social capital describes the number and the quality of relationships between members of society and between individuals and groups within society.
- Disruption of social capital is evidenced by lower interpersonal trust between citizens, and less reciprocity and participation in civic and voluntary associations.
- Lack of social capital is associated with poorer self-rated health.
- Investment in physical infrastructure, public education and tax transfers may generate more social capital than improving interpersonal relationships *per se*.

CHAPTER 16

Social responsibility

Die Medicin ist eine sociale Wissenschaft, und die Politik ist weiter nichts, als Medicin im Grossen.
[Medicine is a social science, and politics is nothing but medicine in the broader perspective.]

Rudolf Virchow, 3 November 1848[23]

DISEASE AND SOCIO-ECONOMIC DEVELOPMENT

The social and political nature of health and disease has been observed by many doctors. One such charismatic doctor was the pathologist Rudolf Virchow who, together with the paediatrician Stephan Friedrich Barez, in 1848 was asked by the Prussian government to investigate an outbreak of 'hunger typhus' (diarrhoea secondary to severe starvation, associated with very high mortality) in the weavers of Upper Silesia. Virchow's conclusions that the epidemic was largely related to the dreadful living conditions, social injustice and poor hygiene regulations and infrastructure were unpopular, and his politically motivated statements that

> ... the proletariat is the result, principally, of the introduction and improvement of machinery ... shall the triumph of human genius lead to nothing more than to make the human race miserable?[24]

incensed the government. Virchow very firmly believed that doctors have the duty to speak out against social injustice and oppression.[23] In 1861 Virchow was elected to the Prussian parliament, and he became an outspoken opponent of Bismarck's hardline policies, and a forceful and effective advocate for social reforms.[24]

Tudor Hart raised similar concerns in his famous 1971 paper *The Inverse Care Law* in relation to the changing conditions in the mining communities in the Wales valleys.[25]

The bleak future now facing mining communities, and others that may suffer similar social dislocation as technical change blunders on without agreed social objectives, cannot be altered by doctors alone; but we do have a duty to draw attention to the need for global costing when it comes to policy decisions on redevelopment or decay of established industrial communities. Such costing would take into account the full social costs and not only those elements of profit and loss traditionally recognised in industry.[25]

HEALTH EFFECTS OF CHILDHOOD ECONOMIC AND SOCIAL PROBLEMS

More than 150 years ago Virchow already alluded to the detrimental health effects of poor socio-economic circumstances. He was confronted with acute illness, still very common in the developing world but rarely seen in the developed world at the beginning of the 21st century. However poor health persists in those growing up in poor socio-economic circumstances.

Several studies have demonstrated the remarkably poorer health status of adults who have grown up in socio-economic disadvantage.[26–32] Those growing up in low socio-economic circumstances have lifelong poorer health on almost all health indicators

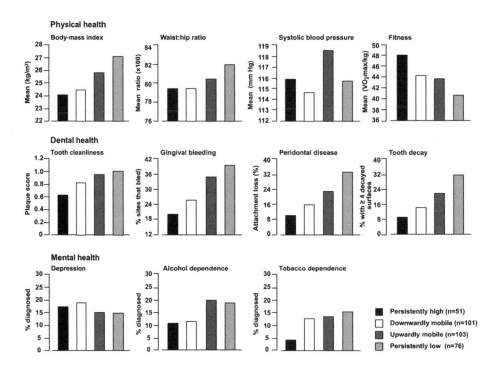

Figure 16.1 Health effects of childhood socio-economic disadvantage. $\dot{V}O_{2max}$: maximum oxygen consumption. (Reproduced from Poulton R, Caspi A, Milne BJ et al. Association between children's experience of socioeconomic disadvantage and adult health: a life-course study. *Lancet.* 2002; **360**: 1640–5,[22] with permission from Elsevier.)

measured – cardiovascular disease,[26,28,31] stroke,[31] respiratory disease and lung cancer,[31] dental health,[26] and mental health[26] and substance abuse.[26] These effects persist even with upward migration in adulthood (*see* Figure 16.1).[26]

Socio-economic circumstances however are not the only factor disadvantaging adult health. Lundberg has shown that besides economic hardship, family life in the first 16 years of life is tremendously important for the future health of children. Growing up in a large family (>4 siblings), a broken family either due to death or divorce, or a home with frequent conflicts or dissension are individually and in combination associated with significantly poorer health and higher mortality (*see* Table 16.1).

TABLE 16.1 Health effects of childhood family situation (from Lundberg O. The impact of childhood living conditions on illness and mortality in adulthood. *Social Science and Medicine.* 1993; **36**: 1047–52,[27] with permission from Elsevier.)

	CHILDHOOD CONDITIONS (ODDS RATIOS)			
MEASURE OF ILL-HEALTH	ECONOMIC HARDSHIP	LARGE FAMILY	BROKEN FAMILY	DISSENSION IN FAMILY
General physical	1.44	1.22	1.35	1.87
Aches and pains	1.49	1.20	1.36	1.97
Circulatory	1.43	1.39	1.64	2.42
Mental	1.83	1.41	1.76	2.75
Mortality over a 3.5-year period	1.16[a]	1.18[a]	1.25[a]	1.46[b]

Indicators of childhood conditions taken separately. Controlling for sex, age, and social class of father. *P* values are highly significant except [a] = not significant; [b] = trend; *n* = 4,216, aged 30–75 years.

HEALTH EFFECTS OF UNEMPLOYMENT

Unemployment, and particularly long-term unemployment amongst the lower socio-economic strata, has become a feature in many developed countries during the late 20th century. General practitioners/family physicians are now confronted regularly with the unemployed as one group of the disadvantaged in our society. We are confronted with their medical, social and mental problems, and their loss of understanding of and belonging to society.

Steinar Westin's work is illuminating and laudable; for a period of 10 years he followed a group of people made unemployed as a consequence of the closure of their workplace, and he documented the impact of that event on their health and health and social services use.[33] The short-term outcomes were not really surprising, most had a higher rate of sick certification during the first year, and they were on average out of work for half of the time during the first two years after losing their job. Over the long term, the gap between the groups persisted, with a large proportion remaining permanently out of work or receiving disability pensions (*see* Figure 16.2).

In addition to the personal direct toll, there are significant indirect health-related effects of unemployment. Controlled follow-up studies have shown an up to 20% increased consultation rate with GPs, an up to 60% increased referral rate to specialist

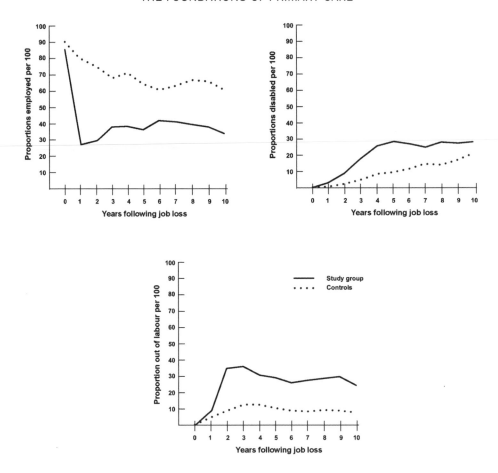

Figure 16.2 Long-term health effects of unemployment. (Adapted from Westin S. The structure of a factory closure: individual responses to job-loss and unemployment in a 10-year controlled follow-up study. *Social Science and Medicine.* 1990; **31**: 1301–11,[29] with permission from Elsevier.)

services, an up to 50% increase in length of sick leave, an up to 300% risk of getting a disability pension, and up to 100% increased risk of dying within 10 years.[34]

In this context it should also be noted that job insecurity and anticipated job loss have substantial subjective health effects and impact on work, social relationships and lifestyle behaviours.[35,36]

How significant these pressures can be may be illustrated by the story of one of my patients, a middle-aged man with more than 20 years' experience in his field and an executive for his branch in his company being put on notice by his young new chief executive officer (CEO) for his personal as well as his department's failure to produce double-digit quarterly growth rates in revenues. He became suicidally depressed by these unrealistic expectations. He subsequently resigned from his position, resulting in the restoration of his health.

The Whitehall II study, involving all London-based office staff working in 20 civil services departments, reported poorer self-perceived health, greater experience of health symptoms in the short term, and a greater number of health problems in the long term. Men are more susceptible to these changes than women.[35] Major downsizing in the workplace, particularly when associated with loss of skill discretion and opportunities in decision making, lead to increased certificated sickness absence – a reliable indicator of health status – deterioration in spousal relationships and increased smoking rates.[36]

HEALTH CONSEQUENCES OF ECONOMIC DECISION MAKING

It is now a common experience that patients perceive difficulties receiving needed care due to underfunded health services. This perception reflects a widely held view that health, and for that matter all other public and community services, are costs without any measurable immediate return, rather than a long-term investment in human and social capital benefiting the economy and society at large.[37]

Steinar Westin explored the shifts in healthcare priorities and healthcare planning since the mid-1980s. He observed:

> Facing the problems of rising costs and the uncontrolled expansion of high tech medical subspecialities, governments and politicians now seem to throw in the towel, finding it easier to abdicate from power and responsibility by leaving the health services to market forces and the expected advantages of professional competition. The irony of the present situation is that while market mechanisms have brought the very expensive American health care system almost to the brink of collapse, it is still the concepts and ideas from market ideologies which now seem to form the blueprint for health care models in large parts of the world.[34]

The consequences of this shift in thinking are particularly stark for the developing world. Again a personal experience reported in the *British Medical Journal* will illustrate this:

> Theresa was waiting for an operation in an African hospital. But as there were so many patients her operation would have to be postponed for another day, or week, or perhaps months. Such postponements are common and the patients quietly wrap their covering sheets around themselves, pick up their medical records, and make their way back to the wards from the waiting area of the operating theatre. Disappointed as most patients are when this happens they are usually hopeful because to have got this far means that they will ultimately get their operation. But Theresa had lost hope and cried in a way that I had never seen an African woman cry before. As I passed I could see the tears just roll down her cheeks as she sat quietly and waited resigned and dignified. During my several working trips to Africa I had seen and heard many women cry in Africa. When the children die the mothers weep and wail and throw themselves on the floor in a way that is very disturbing but Theresa's tears were of a different kind and I was perplexed and curious.
>
> [The medical history revealed that Theresa had an obstructed labour resulting most likely in a stillbirth and a vesicovaginal fistula. She was leaking urine constantly, and required major surgery to repair the injury and to restore her dignity.]

I called one of the nurses over to translate for me and to find some explanation for her weeping. It seemed that Theresa knew that the next day there was to be a government plan to start charging fees for operations. She was a poor woman without money. She thought that as her operation was to be postponed she had lost hope of a cure. All her previous waiting would be in vain and hence the tears.[38]

Clearly health and health care are not commodities. Health services were always intended to *care* for those in need, and seeing a doctor was always regarded as a place of hope when suffering. Destroying hope means destroying health, and destroying health on a large scale jeopardises the survival of whole communities. What we observe here is no different from Virchow's observations 160 years ago, and not surprisingly deserves a similar response.

Under pressure from the International Monetary Fund and the World Bank many powerless African governments have been forced to introduce cuts in health care and education and charge for treatment. Theresa's tears were the human consequences of these policies. No doubt there are many thousands of people like Theresa in Africa. The poorest of the poor are bearing a burden with their lives for the policies of the banks. The debt repayments, the arms trade, and the international unjust trade policies rob Africa of any economic progress. A new brutal and insidious slavery is being perpetuated.[38]

SUMMARY POINTS

- Doctors have an obligation to speak out against social and socio-economic disadvantage.
- Childhood socio-economic disadvantage leads to lifelong poorer health regardless of future economic improvements.
- Unemployment leads to poorer health, and greater use of community resources.
- Even the anticipation of job loss leads to poorer health and greater use of community resources.
- Under-resourcing of primary healthcare services, and making such health services unaffordable, and over-investing in expensive secondary and tertiary disease services, destroys the health of individuals and communities, and ultimately threatens the economic development of communities.
- Neo-liberal policies largely contribute to the demise of the health and well being of individuals and communities.

CHAPTER 17

Health care in societal context

In the consultation, doctor and patient exchange their views about the problem, i.e. they try to construct a *common understanding* of the problem(s) encountered. This exchange does occur in the context of each of the actors' individuality, expectations and experiences. Their interactions are further influenced by the make-up of the local community and the wider society, and hence have an implicit and at times explicit political dimension.

The medical system itself shapes the *social context and its associated expectations of medical care*.[1] This is not necessarily good – as Illich, a most eloquent critic of modern medicine, observed:

> The medical establishment has become a major threat to health. Dependency upon professional health care affects all social relations. In rich countries medical colonization has reached sickening proportions; poor countries are quickly following suit. This process, which I shall call the 'medicalization of life,' deserves articulate political recognition.[39]

In addition the political framework of government as well as medico-political groupings modifies expectations towards the delivery of health care. These differences are particularly obvious comparing the financial models underpinning the healthcare system in the US and the UK. Another major societal driver that has substantially altered the provision of health care is the increasing litigious attitude of patients coupled with the legal system's interpretation of what constitutes reasonable execution of a doctor's duty of care.

HEALTH FINANCING

The financing mechanisms of health care influence the agents in the community in complex ways. For one, health and health care are seen as commodities thus existing for the purpose of maximising profits, for another health and health care are social services and a public good and hence are to be managed based on actual need.[40,41]

These different mental mindsets – and their multiple variations – markedly influence expectations and behaviours of policy makers, health service organisations, and doctors and patients alike. In a market-driven environment, doctors promote their product – delivery of services for all and every ailment – to maximise health expectations and to minimise income losses,[40] by portraying health

> . . . as a state of continued negative reports for hidden disease. Dependence on professional advice for minor ailments is encouraged and is resulting in invalidism and hypochondriasis. Prevention has become a commodity rather than a pattern of behaviour: just another product for sale by the medical entrepreneur.[42]

Elective surgery rates are another example to illustrate this point; the per capita rate of cholecystectomies, prostatectomies and hysterectomies in the US is twice that of the UK. At the same time 15% of US citizens have only access to emergency department care.[40]

The differences in intervention rates and expenditure on health care though have not achieved better population health; in fact within the Organization for Economic Cooperation and Development (OECD), America ranks at the bottom of most health indicators whereas the UK ranks in the top third.[43]

SELF-INTEREST: THE BUSINESS OF MEDICINE

In market-driven healthcare environments, self-interest is at work on several levels. On a personal level the motive of money making alters clinical practice and decision making:

> . . . faster turn-over of patients, shift from continuous to episodic care, increased referral rate to specialists, increased number of tests and increased prescription of drugs.[44]

The impact of personal interest on clinical decision making is particularly noticeable where evidence for a preferred treatment is lacking.[45] The commercialisation and corporatisation of specific services is another example of compromising personal interest over patient interest.[45,46]

The shift in attitudes towards health and health services as readily purchasable perfect commodities, unhappiness with less than expected – even when unrealistic – outcomes has brought into each consultation the fear of medicolegal actions. As a consequence doctors now feel obliged to 'turn every stone' since not doing so may be interpreted as potential evidence of negligence or malpractice.

MARKETING OF HEALTH CARE

Associated with these is the effect of pharmaceutical marketing. It should be clearly evident, despite the fact that the distinctions are often left blurred, that doctors and the pharmaceutical industry have almost diabolical obligations, one to improve the health of patients which at times may involve the use of drugs, the other to maximise profit for their shareholder by turning over product.[47]

The conflict of interest between the medical profession and the pharmaceutical industry is further complicated by their mutual interdependencies. The substantial withdrawal of public funding into health research has made the pharmaceutical industry one of the biggest resource providers of medical research, directing most of their interest into the high-prevalence diseases of Western societies – hypertension, hyperlipidaemia and diabetes. The redefinition of what constitutes hypertension, hyperlipidaemia, raised body mass index and diabetes results in an exponential increase in the prevalence of these condition (*see* Table 17.1), resulting in virtually everyone over the age of 50 having hyperlipidaemia, and more than half of the population being hypertensive.[2,48–50] Westin and Heath have alluded to the fact that there is little evidence that treatment for this group will ever provide any improvement in health outcomes. Figure 17.1 illustrates how underlying assumptions and various statistical methods portray the risk perception for various blood pressure levels.[2,49,51–54]

TABLE 17.1 Gross change in prevalence of disease due to redefinitions (compiled from Schwartz and Woloshin[50])

	% OF POPULATION		CHANGE IN CUT-OFF		NEW CASES	CHANGE %
	OLD	NEW	MMOL/L (MG/DL)	%		
Diabetes	6.20	7.10	8 → 7 (140 → 126)	−10.0	1 681 000	+14
Hypertension	20.6	27.8	160 → 140	−16.7	13 490 000	+35
Hyperlipidaemia	26.4	49.1	6.2 → 5.2 (240 → 200)	−12.5	42 647 000	+86
Body mass index	37.7	53.4	27 → 25	−7.4	29 492 000	+42
Any condition	58.0	75.0			31 880 000	+29

Treating whole populations entails the risk of doing more harm than good. Not only is there a decreasing benefit of treatment with lower risk levels, but this is associated with a corresponding rise in side-effects from treatment, especially for those who are treated with several medications for more than one risk factor. Part of the problem lies in the design of drug trials, which are powered for efficacy endpoints but are grossly underpowered to detect all but major side-effects.[2]

Figure 17.2 shows how increasing medical intervention can lead to harm. There is good evidence to suggest that treatment for high-risk subgroups achieves better health outcomes, and there is equally good evidence that shows that treatment for all other groups does not improve overall function but is associated with more pain, more worry, and more restricted-activity days.[49] The irony is that despite all our efforts the largest number of deaths occurs in those classified as having low risk.

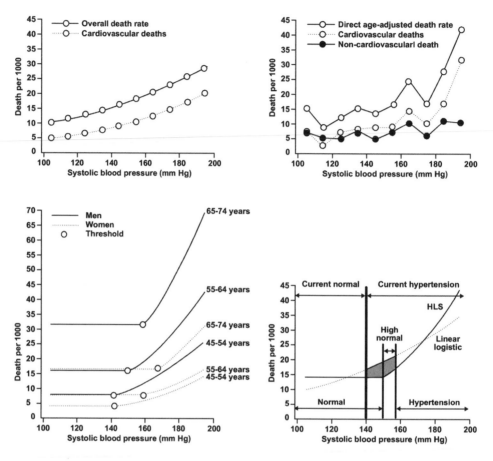

Figure 17.1 Figures from Port outlining the difference in absolute mortality risk from hypertension at various levels of blood pressure. Top left: Framingham age-adjusted mortality rates for men aged 45–74 years related to systolic blood pressure. Rates are obtained form *linear-logistic-regression*, suggesting a *strict linear rise* in risk. Top right: Framingham actual age-adjusted mortality rates for men aged 45–74 years related to systolic blood pressure. Cardiovascular mortality rates are steady up to about 160 mmHg. Bottom left: reduced horizontal-logistic spline (HLS) fits. For 70% of the population the mortality rate for systolic blood pressure remains steady up to the threshold point after which mortality rates rise sharply. Bottom right: superimposing the horizontal-logistic-spline and linear-logistic regression models. Curves are for men aged 55–64 years. The shaded area indicates individuals who may not require any treatment (about 40% of the population). (Reproduced from Port S, Demer L, Jennrich R, Walter D and Garfinkel A. Systolic blood pressure and mortality. *Lancet*. 2000; **355**: 175–80,[50] with permission from Elsevier.)

Taylor summarises, but also reminds us to reconsider the current push for medical intervention in society stating that:

> It is apparent that there is a great deal of bias in favour of more [medical] care, and more costly care, whether or not it helps the patient . . . to use Fuchs' phrase 'medicine should consider the possibility of contributing more by doing less'.[42]

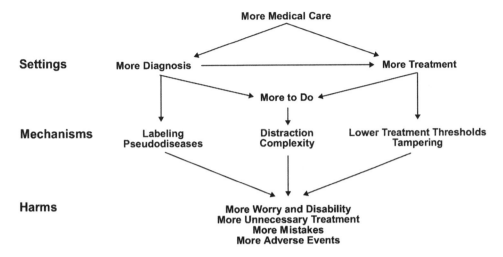

Figure 17.2   How more medical care can cause harm. (From Fisher and Welch,[45] with permission.)

SUMMARY POINTS

- The way we finance health determines how health services are structured and function.
- 'For profit'-oriented health systems produce poorer health at a community level compared to 'not for profit'-oriented systems.
- The intrusion of 'big business' threatens the primacy of the consultation and the healing process.
- Market interests shape and have redefined what constitutes disease.
- The impact of redefinition is an increase in anxiety about health and dying.
- The treatment of 'redefined diseases' has had no meaningful impact on clinical outcomes, and in fact has been shown to cause significant iatrogenic disease and poorer health.
- Doing less often means doing more for the health of individuals and the community at large.

CHAPTER 18

Health inequalities

Health inequalities are a well-recognised phenomenon in most societies, and have been a big political issue in the public health debate. Particularly poor health occurs in most indigenous communities, in poor immigrant and other racially defined communities, and in overcrowded inner-city/urban fringe communities around the world.

It has long been known that the *higher risk of disease and premature death* is *systematically* related to *lower levels of education and income.*[37,55–58] The overall mechanisms causing this increase in morbidity and mortality are not completely understood; however it is postulated that material as well as psychological reasons play an important role.

Health inequality has been correlated to socio-economic status. At the individual level, socio-economic status regardless of whether it is measured by occupation, education or household income, is strongly correlated with an individual's health. Daly described the complex relationship as

> . . . the correlation between SES [socio-economic status] and health is invariably positive, and is often best described as a continuous but nonlinear 'gradient': large improvements in health are associated with incremental gains in SES among populations at the lower end of the socioeconomic scale, whereas smaller health gains are associated with increments in SES among groups situated at higher levels of the scale.[58]

The socio-economic status is invariably associated with the infrastructure and opportunities of a neighbourhood, and the social cohesion or tension within.

INCOME INEQUALITY

Poverty is the mother of all disease.

Johann Peter Frank, 1790[59]

Income inequality reflects structural characteristics of the economy, political decisions regarding welfare and Social Security payments, and family demographic characteristics.[58] Specific factors affecting an individual's income level include: general employment opportunities; technological change altering the workplace; increased monetary reward for those with higher education or skills; the expected rate of return on capital investment; level of welfare payments and tax policies; policies affecting family size and family support.

Daly described two related propositions linking income inequality and health:

> First, an inequitable income distribution may be associated with a set of economic, political, social, and institutional processes that reflect a systematic underinvestment in human, physical, health, and social infrastructure. This underinvestment has possible consequences for both poor and middle-class individuals and thus represents a *material dimension* to the inequality – health link.
>
> Second, inequitable income distribution may directly affect people's perceptions of their social environment, which may in turn have an impact on their health. This constitutes a *psychological dimension* to the relation between inequality and health. The material and psychological strands are linked to the extent that perceptions of inequality are based on material conditions.[58]

Daly further observed a political dimension: 'political units' that allow higher income inequality in their jurisdiction are less likely to support the provision of human, physical, cultural, civic, and health resource, and that communities with high income inequality may be less equitable in their support of education, affordable housing, good infrastructure and environmental protection. These mechanisms would support the interrelated nature of material and psychological dimensions of income inequality on health.

The net effect of income inequality (as measured by the Robin Hood Index) on mortality is substantial; a 1% rise in income inequality (adjusted for poverty) is related to an age-adjusted increase in total mortality of 21.7 deaths per 100 000.[55] The level of income inequality within communities, independent of the absolute income level of an individual, strongly correlates with self-perceived health (*see* Figure 18.1).[37] Also, self-perceived health very strongly correlates with future mortality.[60]

HOW INCOME INEQUALITY MAY CAUSE POOR HEALTH

Three plausible mechanisms have been identified that link income inequality to poor health: disinvestment in human capital, erosion of social capital, and directly due to stressful social comparisons.[37]

Underinvestment in education has been shown to occur in communities with high income inequality, resulting in poorer educational outcomes and higher school dropouts, leading to diminished life opportunities for the poor.[37] Krugman suggests that the rising income inequality leads to a divergence of interests between the rich and the poor. He states that (in the US):

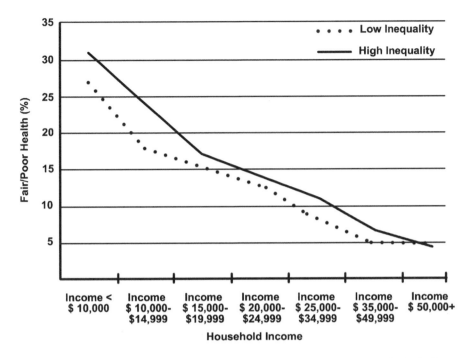

Figure 18.1 The effect of income inequality on self-rated health according to levels of individual income and levels of income inequality. (Reproduced from Kawachi I and Kennedy B. Income inequality and health: pathways and mechanisms. *Health Services Research.* 1999; **34**: 215–27,[33] with permission from Blackwell Publishing.)

A family at the 95th percentile pays a lot more in taxes than a family at the 50th, but it does not receive a correspondingly higher benefit from public services, such as education. The greater the income gap, the greater the disparity in interests. This translates, because of the clout of the elite, into a constant pressure for lower taxes and reduced public services.[61]

Kawachi *et al.*,[16] in an ecological study, showed that disinvestment in social capital is one of the possible pathways by which income inequality produces detrimental effects on population mortality. Table 18.1 indicates the magnitude of impact associated with a 1% change in four different indicators of social capital, e.g. a 1% decline in engagement with voluntary groups is associated with an age-adjusted rise in total mortality of 83.17 per 100 000. Loss of social trust also negatively impacts on infant mortality, heart disease and malignancies.

TABLE 18.1 The effects of a 1% change in social capital indicators on age-adjusted health (compiled from Kawachi et al.[16])

	LACK OF FAIRNESS[a]		MISTRUST[b]		LACK OF HELPFULNESS[c]		VOLUNTARY GROUP MEMBERSHIP	
	CHANGE IN NO OF DEATHS/100 000	VARIANCE[d]	CHANGE IN NO OF DEATHS/100 000	VARIANCE[d]	CHANGE IN NO OF DEATHS/100 000	VARIANCE[d]	CHANGE IN NO OF DEATHS/100 000	VARIANCE[d]
Total mortality								
unadjusted	6.71	58	5.32	61	7.01	49	-83.17	22
adjusted for poverty	5.61	63	4.54	64	5.69	50	-66.75	45
Infant mortality								
unadjusted	0.12	42	0.08	30	0.14	46	[-0.98]	[5]
adjusted for poverty	0.10	43	0.06	32	0.13	42	[-0.67]	[21]
Heart disease								
unadjusted	1.32	15	(0.98)	(14)	(1.50)	(15)	-25.99	16
adjusted for poverty	1.08	15	(0.78)	(13)	(1.29)	(14)	-23.03	20
Malignant neoplasms								
unadjusted	0.95	20	0.84	27	(0.76)	(8)	-20.32	25
adjusted for poverty	1.03	18	0.97	26	(0.86)	(6)	-19.81	23
Cerebrovascular disease								
unadjusted	[0.48]	[16]	0.42	21	[0.54]	[16]	[-2.44]	[1]
adjusted for poverty	[0.33]	[20]	0.97	23	[0.35]	[17]	[-0.71]	[13]
Unintentional injuries								
unadjusted	0.51	22	[0.42]	[26]	[0.69]	[32]	[-2.47]	[1]
adjusted for poverty	0.17	57	[0.14]	[58]	[0.21]	[57]	[0.58]	[55]

a Measured by the percentage of people responding: 'Most people would try to take advantage of you if they got the chance'.

b Measured by the percentage of people responding: 'You can't be too careful in dealing with people'.

c Measured by the percentage of people responding: 'People mostly look out for themselves'.

d % variance in the regression model (explanatory power).

Figures in parentheses indicate borderline significance, figures in square brackets indicate non-significance.

At an ecological level these data suggest that socially isolated people could potentially benefit from living in a neighbourhood with high social capital, and conversely, that living in a neighbourhood with poor social capital negatively impacts on an individual's health regardless of their own resources.

However, on a societal level, the predominance of the market focus has led to a neglect of most types of public goods, and in particular the production of social capital.[51] The implications for the coherence of society are bleak.

> What our empirical data do support is that the growing gap between the rich and the poor affects the social organization of communities and that the resulting damage to the social fabric may have profound implications for the public's health.[55]

CONSEQUENCES OF INCOME INEQUALITY

Two aspects need to be considered, absolute and relative income inequality. The relative gap between the well off and the poor in a community, rather than the absolute standard of living of the poor, appear to be strongly related to overall mortality and disease-specific mortality (infant mortality, heart disease, malignancy, homicide), and to a somewhat smaller degree to potentially treatable disease (infectious diseases, tuberculosis, hypertension).[55,57]

Overall mortality risk is strongly predicted by a person's residence being in a recognised poverty neighbourhood, and the risk is independent of the person's individual- and family-level socio-economic status.[57,58]

Kawachi and co-workers calculated that a 1% increase in income inequality is associated with an excess mortality of 21.7 deaths per 100 000, and further estimated that lowering the income inequality in the US to that of the UK, the age-adjusted mortality from coronary heart disease could be lowered by 25% (from 183 to 139 per 100 000), and overall mortality by 7%, assuming a causal relationship.[55,62] They concluded that the alleviation of poverty must be a policy priority for the US.

Income distribution can be seen as a proxy indicator for social disadvantage through underinvestment in human capital, including public education and accessible health care.[51] Policy initiatives like comprehensive welfare and redistributive policies of Northern European states have demonstrated their effects on evening out some of the negative effects of social disadvantage.[56]

SUMMARY POINTS

- Higher risk of disease and premature death are systematically related to lower levels of education and income.
- Poverty is the mother of all disease.
- The greater the income inequality within a community, the poorer is the health of the lower income stratum.
- A small reduction in income inequality leads to a marked improvement in age-adjusted all-cause mortality.
- Relative income inequality is a more important factor of poor health than the absolute level of income.

CHAPTER 19

Emerging patterns

What is accepted is no longer valid, what is valid is not yet accepted.

Jamshid Gharajedaghi

The surgery is the microcosm of society. Doctors, in every consultation, are confronted with the great, the ordinary and the ugly in society. Our privileged position gives us a deep insight into the effects of societal activity on the health of our patients, makes us a particularly powerful bearer of the conscience of society, and demands that we speak out against all forms of societal abuse, an insight no more clearly articulated than by Virchow.

A clear pattern emerges: social and societal activities impact greatly, though at times subtly, on the health of our patients. One aspect of this pattern is the family one is born into – providing economic as well as emotional privileges – another the make-up and the resources available in the local community – social capital, community infrastructure, education and work opportunities – and yet another society's shaping of health, illness and disease and the associated commitment to equitable and affordable health care to its citizens (*see* Figure 19.1).

Healthy individuals live in healthy societies, and vice versa; sick individuals live in sick societies. Lessons need to be learnt from this simple and straightforward truism.

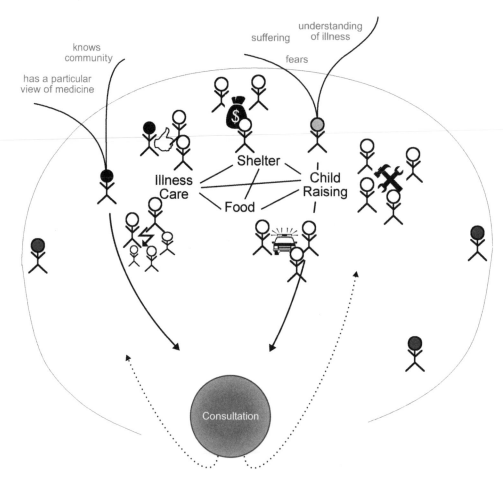

Figure 19.1 Social and societal factors impacting on health. Societal reality is reflected overtly in the consultation. Factors affecting the wellbeing of individuals and society include, amongst others, the composition and functioning of families, work opportunities and security, social infrastructure, economic ideology, and the degree of cohesion and integration between members of the community.

REFERENCES

1 Rosenberg C. Disease in history: frames and framers. *Milbank Quarterly.* 1989; **67**(Suppl 1): 1–15.

2 Westin S and Heath I. Thresholds for normal blood pressure and serum cholesterol. *British Medical Journal.* 2005; **330**: 1461–2.

3 Thabo Mbeki. Opening Speech at the 13th International AIDS Conference, 9 July 2000, Durban. www.anc.org.za/ancdocs/history/mbeki/2000/tm0709.html (accessed 5 July 2006).

4 Jordi Casabona. Opening Speech at the 14th International AIDS Conference, 7 July 2002, Durban. www.kaisernetwork.org/aids2002/transcript/transcript_webcast_08_b.html (accessed 5 July 2006).

5 Thaksin Shinawatra. Opening Speech at the 15th International AIDS Conference, 11 July 2004, Bangkok. www.thaigov.go.th/news/speech/thaksin/sp11Jul04-2.htm (accessed 5 July 2006).

6 Glouberman S and Zimmerman B. *Complicated and Complex Systems: what would successful reform of medicare look like?*: Discussion paper No 8. Ottawa: Commission on the Future of Health Care in Canada, 2002.

7 Daly J and McDonald I. *The Social Impact of Echocardiography*. Canberra: Australian Institute of Health and Welfare, 1993.

8 Greenhalgh T and Hurwitz B. Narrative based medicine: why study narrative? *British Medical Journal*. 1999; **318**: 48–50.

9 Fredriksen S. Instrumental colonisation in modern medicine. *Medicine, Health Care and Philosophy*. 2003; **6**: 287–96.

10 Green L, Fryer G, Yawn B, Lanier D and Dovey S. The ecology of medical care revisited. *New England Journal of Medicine*. 2001; **344**: 2021–5.

11 Turnberg L. Science, society and the perplexed physician. *Journal of the Royal College of Physicians of London*. 2000; **34**: 569–75.

12 Bullen P and Onyx J. *Measuring Social Capital in Five Communities in NSW – A Practitioners' Guide*. Coogee, Australia: Management Alternatives Pty, 1998.

13 Grootaert C. *Social Capital: the missing link?* **Social Capital** Initiative Working Paper No. 3, Washington DC: The World Bank. www.siteresources.worldbank.org/INTSOCIALCAPITAL/Resources/Social-Capital-Initiative-Working-Paper-Series/SCI-WPS-03.pdf

14 Putman R. The prosperous community. Social capital and public life. *American Prospect*. 1993; **13**: 35–42.

15 Coleman J. Social capital in the creation of human capital. *American Journal of Sociology*. 1988; **94**(Suppl): S95–S120.

16 North D. *Institutions, Institutional Change and Economic Performance*. New York: Cambridge University Press, 1990.

17 Olson M. *The Rise and Decline of Nations: economic growth, stagflation, and social rigidities*. New Haven: Yale University Press, 1982.

18 Szreter S and Woolcock M. Health by association? Social capital, social theory, and the political economy of public health. *International Journal of Epidemiology*. 2004; **33**: 650–67.

19 Kavanagh AM, Turrell G and Subramanian SV. Does area-based social capital matter for the health of Australians? A multilevel analysis of self-rated health in Tasmania. *International Journal of Epidemiology*. 2006; **35**: 607–13.

20 Kawachi I, Kennedy B, Lochner K and Prothrow-Stith D. Social capital, income inequality, and mortality. *American Journal of Public Health*. 1997; **87**: 1491–8.

21 Kawachi I, Kim D, Coutts A and Subramanian SV. Commentary: Reconciling the three accounts of social capital. *International Journal of Epidemiology*. 2004; **33**: 682–90.

22 Poortinga W. Social relations or social capital? Individual and community health effects of bonding social capital. *Social Science and Medicine*. 2006; **63**: 255–70.

23 Bauer A. 'Die Medicin ist eine sociale Wissenschaft' – Rudolf Virchow (1821–1902) als Pathologe, Politiker und Publizist. *Medicine – Bibliothek – Information*. 2005; **5**: 16–20.

24 *Who Named It? Rudolf Ludwig Karl Virchow*. www.whonamedit.com/doctor.cfm/912.html (accessed 5 July 2006).

25 Hart J. The Inverse Care Law. *Lancet*. 1971; **I**: 405–12.

26 Poulton R, Caspi A, Milne BJ *et al*. Association between children's experience of socioeconomic disadvantage and adult health: a life-course study. *Lancet*. 2002; **360**: 1640–5.

27 Lundberg O. The impact of childhood living conditions on illness and mortality in adulthood. *Social Science and Medicine*. 1993; **36**: 1047–52.

28 Brunner E, Shipley M, Blane D, Smith G and Marmot M. When does cardiovascular risk start? Past and present socioeconomic circumstances and risk factors in adulthood. *Journal of Epidemiology and Community Health*. 1999; **53**: 757–64.

29 Bosma H, van de Mheen HD and Mackenbach JP. Social class in childhood and general health in adulthood: questionnaire study of contribution of psychological attributes. *British Medical Journal*. 1999; **318**: 18–22.

30 Laaksonen M, Rahkonen O, Martikainen P and Lahelma E. Socioeconomic position and self-rated health: the contribution of childhood socioeconomic circumstances, adult socioeconomic status, and material resources. *American Journal of Public Health*. 2005; **95**: 1403–9.

31 Power C, Hyppönen E and Davey Smith G. Socioeconomic position in childhood and early adult life and risk of mortality: a prospective study of the mothers of the 1958 British birth cohort. *American Journal of Public Health*. 2005; **95**: 1396–402.

32 Fone D, Jones A, Watkins J *et al*. Using local authority data for action on health inequalities: the Caerphilly Health and Social Needs Study. *British Journal of General Practice*. 2002; **52**: 799–804.

33 Westin S. The structure of a factory closure: individual responses to job-loss and unemployment in a 10-year controlled follow-up study. *Social Science and Medicine*. 1990; **31**: 1301–11.

34 Westin S. The market is a strange creature: family medicine meeting the challenges of the changing political and socioeconomic structure. *Family Practice*. 1995; **12**: 394–401.

35 Ferrie J, Shipley M, Marmot M, Stansfeld S and Smith G. Health effects of anticipation of job change and non-employment: longitudinal data from the Whitehall II study. *British Medical Journal*. 1995; **311**: 1264–9.

36 Kivimäki M, Vahtera J, Pentti J and Ferrie J. Factors underlying the effect of organisational downsizing on health of employees: longitudinal cohort study. *British Medical Journal*. 2000; **320**: 971–5.

37 Kawachi I and Kennedy B. Income inequality and health: pathways and mechanisms. *Health Services Research*. 1999; **34**: 215–27.

38 Towey R. A memorable patient. An African woman weeps. *British Medical Journal*. 1995; **310**: 1104.

39 Illich I. *Limits to Medicine. Medical Nemesis: the expropriation of health*. London: Marion Boyars Book, 1976.

40 Hart J. Expectations of health care: promoted, managed or shared? *Health Expectations*. 1998; **1**: 3–13.

41 Davies H and Marshall M. UK and US health-care systems: divided by more than a common language. *Lancet*. 2000; **355**: 336.

42 Taylor R. *Medicine Out of Control*. Melbourne: Sun Books, 1979.

43 Starfield B. Is US health really the best in the World? *Journal of the American Medical Association*. 2000; **284**: 483–5.

44 Fugelli P. Clinical practice: between Aristotle and Cochrane. *Schweizerische Medizinische Wochenschrift*. 1998; **128**: 184–8.

45 Moynihan R. Too much medicine? The business of health and its risks for you. *Too much Medicine*. ABC-Television, 1998. http://abc.net.au/science/slab/medicine/default.htm (accessed 5 July 2006).

46 Ewig S. Was ist ein guter Arzt? *Frankfurter Allgemeine Sonntagszeitung*. 2006; **7 May**: 73–4.

47 PLoS Medicine. Disease mongering. *PLoS Medicine*. 2006; **3**(4). http://collections.plos.org/diseasemongering-2006.php (accessed 5 July 2006).

48 Meador C. The art and science of nondisease. *New England Journal of Medicine*. 1965; **272**: 92–5.

49 Fisher E and Welch H. Avoiding the unintended consequences of growth in medical care. How might more be worse? *Journal of the American Medical Association*. 1999; **281**: 446–53.

50 Schwartz L and Woloshin S. Changing disease definitions: implications for disease prevalence. *Effective Clinical Practice*. 1999; **2**: 76–85.

51 Law M and Wald N. Risk factor thresholds: their existence under scrutiny. *British Medical Journal*. 2002; **324**: 1570–6.

52 Davey Smith G, Song F and Sheldon T. Cholesterol lowering and mortality: the importance of considering initial level of risk. *British Medical Journal*. 1993; **306**: 1367–73.

53 Hetlevik I, Holmen J and Krüger Ø. Implementing clinical guidelines in the treatment of hypertension in general practice. *Scandinavian Journal of Primary Health Care*. 1999; **17**: 35–40.

54 Port S, Demer L, Jennrich R, Walter D and Garfinkel A. Systolic blood pressure and mortality. *Lancet*. 2000; **355**: 175–80.

55 Kennedy B, Kawachi I and Prothrow-Stith D. Income distribution and mortality: cross sectional ecological study of the Robin Hood index in the United States. *British Medical Journal*. 1996; **312**: 1004–7.

56 Mackenbach J and Hawden-Chapman P. New perspectives on socioeconomic inequalities in health. *Perspectives in Biology and Medicine*. 2003; **46**: 428–44.

57 Shi L, Starfield B, Kennedy B and Kawachi I. Income inequality; primary care, and health indicators. *Journal of Family Practice*. 1999; **48**: 275–84.

58 Daly M, Duncan G, Kaplan G and Lynch J. Macro-to micro links in the relation between income inequality and mortality. *Milbank Quarterly*. 1998; **76**: 315–39.

59 Frank JP. The people's misery: mother of diseases. *Bulletin of History in Medicine*. 1941; **9**: 81–100.

60 Idler E and Benyamini Y. Self-rated health and mortality: a review of twenty-seven community studies. *Journal of Health and Social Behaviour*. 1997; **38**: 21–37.

61 Krugman P. The spiral of inequality. *Mother Jones*. 1996; **November/December**: 44–49. www.motherjones.com/news/feature/1996/11/krugman.html (accessed 5 July 2006).

62 Kawachi I and Kennedy BP. The relationship of income inequality to mortality: does the choice of indicator matter? *Social Science and Medicine*. 1997; **45**: 1121–7.

History	Philosophy	The Practice of Medicine	Social	Primary Care
Social Construct of Health Public Health Infrastructure	Husserl	Personal Relationship Phronesis Continuity of Care Care Co-ordination Quality of Life	Social Capital	Common Goal Integrated BUT Diverse Solutions
Shaman/Medicine Man Hippocrates of Cos Care for the Whole Patient	Pellegrino		Income Inequality	
	Cynefin Knowledge Model			
Broad Education Apprenticeship Model of Learning	Cartesian Dualism ←→ Complexity		Employment	
Knowledge of Disease School of Cnidus	Popper	Science & Technology	Access	Personal Health Gain

SECTION FIVE

Medicine in the community: towards primary care

Co-author: Carmel Martin MBBS MSC PhD FRACGP MRCGP FAFPHM, A/Prof of Family Medicine, Northern Ontario Medical School, Sudbury, Canada

> And then they have that way, nowadays, of sending you off to a specialist: 'I can only diagnose your trouble,' a doctor will tell you, 'but if you go to see such and such a specialist. He'll know how to cure it.' I tell you, the old doctor who could cure you of every illness has all but vanished and you find nothing but specialists these days, and they even advertise in newspapers.
>
> *Dostoevsky* – The Brothers Karamazov[1]

> Managers are not confronted with problems that are independent of each other, but with dynamic situations that consist of changing problems that interact with each other. I call such situations messes . . . managers do not solve problems: they manage messes.
>
> *Russ Ackoff*[2]

Could Dostoevsky really have foreshadowed the developments of medical practice? Well, we will never know for sure, but his description certainly is close to the experiences of both doctors and patients at the beginning of the 21st century.

181

Two disparate but interconnected issues influence the future developments of the healthcare system – the Cartesian-based compartmentalisation of the body has shaped a specialist orientated health service; the current health system will continue to influence the conceptualisations and practices of medicine in the evolving primary care oriented one.

As the first four sections have demonstrated, history is living on in medicine. The *'want and need'* for receiving medical care when feeling ill is a constant feature of all human societies, as is the need to have an *ongoing trusting and personal relationship with the doctor*, and the need to *make sense out of the illness experience*. The effectiveness of the personal therapeutic relationship is central to healing, and is firmly embedded in modern societies despite the scientific and technological advances of disease-based care.

Throughout the first four sections I have hinted at the complex relationships and interactions of the various phenomena described. This section presents a unifying model of primary care as a complex adaptive system. This model emerged out of the ongoing collaboration between Carmel Martin and myself, thus we have jointly written the following two chapters.

The first chapter in this section describes the concepts of primary (health) care and elaborates how primary care can deliver improved and more equitable care to the community.

The second chapter examines primary care and its changing nature. We have developed the healthcare vortex as a metaphor to conceptualise the different agendas and layers of the 'healthcare' system. Systems are driven by core values; we make the case that the core value of medical care is the improvement of *personal health*, the value inherent and constant since the beginnings of medicine, and that the achievement of *personal health* depends on an *ongoing personal healing relationship with the doctor*.

The calls for ongoing health system reform are here to stay. The challenge for the managers of the reform process remains, how to create the *space of possibilities* in which to allow all of the different perspectives on health care to be explored constructively in light of its core value. The evidence provided here and synthesised in the healthcare vortex should provide a foundation for this process.

CHAPTER 20

Primary care

> A human being is part of a whole, the 'universe'. Our task must be to free our-
> selves from the delusion of separateness.
>
> *Albert Einstein*

The terms 'primary care' and 'primary health centre' date back to the 1920s. A UK White Paper, the Dawson Report, suggested that primary health centres would become the hub for regionalised health services for a community.[3] The health services model at that time was largely based around the single-handed GP in the community who provided both community-based and hospital-based care to their patients.

GPs/family physicians have been the primary sources of medical care for many centuries, though many minor ailments were always treated with house remedies or by non-medical healthcare providers (in today's terms: allied healthcare providers and alternative practitioners).

Only since the 1960s has specialisation, and since the 1980s subspecialisation, become a prominent feature in health care. This move has not only depleted the number but also has led to a loss of self-esteem and a sense of devaluation of generalist physicians.[4] The structure of the medical education process, being tertiary centre-based, constantly promotes a superiority notion of the specialist teacher's in-depth technical knowledge over the generalist's broad contextual knowledge. Such comments on the one hand expose a mindset of *medicine as a technical endeavour*, on the other negate the *reality of the nature of illness* in the community. Associated with the latter goes a disregard of a uniquely different knowledge and skills set, one that allows community physicians to deal with up to 99% of all illness in the general population.[5]

THE FOUNDATIONS OF PRIMARY CARE

In 1920 Dawson introduced the term 'primary care'[3] as part of the social health movement to address health disparities and the increasing complexities of healthcare delivery.[3] These were the same concerns that in 1978 led to the Alma-Ata declaration (*see* Appendix) and the WHO's adoption and promulgation of the term 'primary health care'. The primary care strategy set out to integrate health promotion and disease prevention, and to foster co-ordinated care for those with complex disease. This vision was seen as the means to address the widespread health inequalities in many communities.[6]

Explicit in the move to primary (health) care is the concept of social justice, and equity of access to care. Implicitly the move entails varying concepts of service restructuring, including centralisation or co-ordination of care, division of labour among the different healthcare providers, and shifting the workforce and its skill-mix to fit the perception of care requiring an 'increasingly complex disease focus'.

It always was envisaged that physicians co-ordinate health care through integration and sharing of needed care with other healthcare providers in the community. Dawson envisaged that this would be achieved through a well-thought out organisational structure that would be flexible enough to respond to unique local conditions:

> The general availability of medical services can only be effected by new and extended organisation, distributed according to the needs of the community. This organisation is needed on grounds of efficiency and cost, and is necessary alike in the interest of the public and of the medical profession. Measures for dealing with health and disease become, with increasing knowledge, more complex, and, therefore, less within the power of the individual to provide, but rather require combined efforts. Such combined efforts to yield the best results must be located in the same institution.[7]

The Dawson Report however did not seek to displace GPs/family physicians and their surgeries close to the people and their homes, nor did it suggest any form of substitution for their care:

> The custom whereby each general practitioner has his consulting rooms at his own house should, under ordinary circumstances, continue, but where, as in certain congested areas, it is impossible for a doctor to provide adequate accommodation at his own expense, it should be possible, if the public interest demanded it, for the Health Authority to provide such accommodation at the Primary Health Centre, or elsewhere, on such terms as are reasonable, and after previous consultation with a Local Medical Advisory Council. Where local conditions, and medical opinion, favoured the plan, collective surgeries might with advantage be tried, either attached to a primary health centre, or set up elsewhere.[7]

A DEFINITION FOR THE 21ST CENTURY

A modern interpretation of the distinctions between primary health care and primary care has been articulated by Kelleher:

> *Primary health care (PHC)* incorporates personal care with health promotion, the prevention of illness and community development. The philosophy of PHC includes the interconnecting principles of equity, access, empowerment, community self-

determination and intersectoral collaboration. It encompasses an understanding of the social, economic, cultural and political determinants of health.

Primary care is more clinically focused, and can be considered a sub-component of the broader primary healthcare system. Primary care is considered health care provided by a medical professional which is a [patient's] first point of entry into the health system. Primary care is practised widely in nursing and allied health, but predominately in general practice.[8]

The most recent revisitation of this vision of socially responsible medicine and health care continues to adhere to the visions of Dawson and Alma-Ata but encompasses a broader vision for both developed and developing countries (Pan American Health Organization (PAHO)/WHO, 2005) (*see* Box 20.1).[9]

BOX 20.1 The aims of primary health care: Declaration of Montevideo

Regional declaration on the new orientations for primary health care (Declaration of Montevideo) (compiled from reference 9).
1 Commitment to facilitate social inclusion and equity in health.
2 Recognition of the critical roles of both the individual and the community in the development of primary health care (PHC)-based systems.
3 Orientation toward health promotion and comprehensive and integrated care.
4 Development of intersectoral work.
5 Orientation toward quality of care and patient safety.
6 Strengthening of human resources in health.
7 Establishment of structural conditions that allow PHC renewal.
8 Guarantee of financial sustainability.
9 Research and development and appropriate technology.
10 Network strengthening and partnerships of international co-operation in support of PHC.

CARE NEEDS DEPEND ON THE UNDERLYING ILLNESS

The shifting morbidity burden (*see* Table 20.1) associated with the aging of the population has led to a shift in care needs. To maintain the holistic nature of health care requires an expansion, not substitution of our essential role, in the services to our patients. We share with our patients the journey into illness. Part of our care includes linking their evolving specific care needs to those medical and allied healthcare professionals with the relevant specific expertise.

Figure 20.1 illustrates the patterns of decline in an aging population. Most elderly remain healthy, and only 10% will suffer from chronic illnesses that require constant and multidimensional care.

A well-functioning primary healthcare system must be able to simultaneously and equitably address the maintenance of wellness and the care of the different degrees of chronic illness. In particular the system must have the capacity to address the distinctive needs associated with the trajectories of cancer, organ failure and frailty.

TABLE 20.1 Ten leading sources of the global burden of disease, 1990 and 2020 (Source: Murray[10])

RANK	1990 DISEASE OR INJURY	2020 DISEASE OR INJURY
1	Lower respiratory infection	Ischaemic heart disease
2	Diarrhoeal diseases	Unipolar major depression
3	Conditions arising during the perinatal period	Road traffic accidents
4	Unipolar major depression	Cerbrovascular diseases
5	Ischaemic heart disease	Chronic obstructive pulmonary disease
6	Cerbrovascular diseases	Lower respiratory infection
7	Tuberculosis	Tuberculosis
8	Measles	War
9	Road traffic accidents	Diarrhoeal diseases
10	Congenital anomalies	HIV/AIDS

CARE CO-ORDINATION

People with serious acute or chronic illness or other 'non-medical' life problems may have periods where they are overwhelmed by their illness or circumstances. This is most likely to occur at periods of transition such as at the time of diagnosis, transition to the terminal stage of illness, or at the time of events like job loss or relationship break-up. These are the times of considerable somato-psycho-socio-semiotic needs requiring a wide range of support to co-ordinate the required care of the physical, emotional, social and sense-making domains.

A comprehensive and co-ordinated approach to the complex care needs supports a patient's trajectory through the different care environments ranging from acute hospital to ongoing community care. Important aspects of this 'whole person care' approach include attention to such issues as health, welfare, justice, employment and education problems (*see* Box 20.2).[12]

BOX 20.2 People's support needs to enable complex care (reproduced and adapted from Martin,[12] with permission)

People with chronic illness or serious acute conditions, particularly those in crisis with complex care needs, require increased support to cope and to become resourceful self managers.[13] The types of support[14] include:

■ *informational support*: providing and delivering patient and carer education about the disease and/or illness, treatment, prevention, and access to additional information, including the internet

■ *decisional support* at the time of making choices when there is, or is not a clear-cut decision to be made, e.g. type of surgery for breast cancer

■ *social support*: understanding and utilising the skills of the carer, family network, friends and peers who are going through similar experiences

■ *emotional support*: being empathic and communicating effectively on a range of topics which include intimate and emotional issues

■ *appraisal support*: giving appropriate and timely feedback

- *practical support*: navigating through complex treatment and services, and addressing issues such as finances, transportation, housing, and overall welfare
- *personal rapport, engagement and friendship*
- *spiritual support*
- *nutritional information and support*
- *recovery support*: meanings and expectations on and about the recovery process (duration, degree of impairment, stages of recovery)
- *transitions support*: from acute to chronic, chronic to end-stage, exacerbations and remissions

Care for chronic illness or serious acute conditions benefits from comprehensive and multifaceted health service delivery. Key elements of chronic illness management include:[15,16]

- personnel and care processes to support proactive care, including case management and scheduling/co-ordination of visits and follow-up

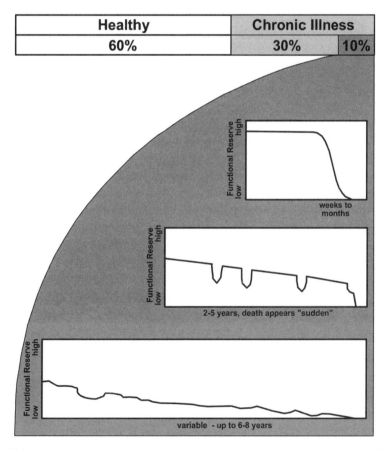

Figure 20.1 Patterns of decline in an ageing population. (Reprinted from Lynn J and Adamson D. *Living Well at the End of Life. Adapting health care to serious chronic illness in old age.* Santa Monica, CA: Rand Health, 2003,[9] with permission from Rand Corporation.)

- decision support for providers, including guidelines/protocols
- information systems to ensure access to timely and relevant information
- patient responsibility and support for self-management
- community resources to inform and support patients
- system support for chronic illness care.

QUALITY OF LIFE AND SELF-RATED HEALTH

Quality of life and self-rated health are not only good indicators for individual health, but would appear to also be useful indicators of the health of communities. External factors that emerge as consistently impacting on quality of life and self-rated health would be those that require a *community development response*, a strategy that has been accepted to be part of the primary healthcare concept.

Quality of life describes the *patient's personal perception* of not only his health status but also all other 'environmental' circumstances that impact on his life. The response to the question 'How do you rate the quality of your life?' provides insight into the patient's current experience of his quality of life. The interdependence of physical and other life circumstances on quality of life is illustrated by the following two scenarios:

> With an appropriate environment, support, and emotional condition, some persons may regard their quality of life as excellent, despite substantial medical and physical infirmities.

> Other persons, despite apparently excellent health, may think their quality of life is poor, because of social, interpersonal, intrapersonal, financial, or other problems.[17]

Self-rated health is a related but different concept to quality of life. 'How do you rate your health – excellent, very good, good, fair or poor' seeks an individual's perception of his health, irrespective of disease, diagnoses, or other factors. Adjusting the self-rated health response for these attributes shows that – in cohort studies – it is an independent predictor of mortality.[18] Poor self-rated health is associated with an up to 93.5 times greater mortality risk compared to those in excellent health.[18]

The meaning of the patient's expressed perceptions and experiences of health and quality of life may not be clear to the physician, particularly if they are sufficiently different from his own judgement. Further exploration may be required – in medical, physical, emotional, spiritual, social, financial, occupational and other domains.[17]

WHAT DOES PRIMARY (HEALTH) CARE OFFER GOVERNMENTS, THE PUBLIC AND PATIENTS?

Governments in the industrialised world view primary care as a solution to the escalating costs of their healthcare systems. However, the pressure to achieve better expenditure control and/or greater productivity and economic efficiency needs to be balanced against the deeply rooted moral imperatives to maintain universal access to necessary care, and to improve the equity with which services are distributed across social classes.[19] Governments in the developing world view primary care as the best approach to achieve better global health. In 2003 the WHO concluded:

Both the Millennium Development Goals (MDGs) and the Report of the Commission on Macroeconomics and Health recommend and assume extensive new financial inputs to health care. There is a general move towards service systems based on and led by PHC with the realization that its principles – such as universal access and coverage, its role as the site of first contact, community participation, integration of service are relevant to all populations and communities – maximize health development and respond to the patterns of disease, in demographic profiles and in socioeconomic environments that present massive new challenges to PHC.[20]

While primary (health) care espouses whole-person comprehensive and patient-centred care, there are increasing centralised pressures and incentives around *disease* targets and some narrowly defined views of success.[9,21,22] Yet we have previously demonstrated that there are striking discontinuities and differences between health and disease, all of which have long been understood (and repeatedly debated) throughout the history of medicine.

With regard to health care for people with chronic disease, general practice/family medicine is caught in a bind. Technology and specialism-oriented services have led to the development of a multidisciplinary workforce scattered across different healthcare settings and sectors. Still, the lessons from e.g. HIV/AIDS clearly indicate the need to take policy back to the *generalist multiskilled individual practitioner* bonded in a therapeutic alliance with the patient and his disease.

> . . . a patient may need to see as many as five different providers, highlighting the need for multiskilled providers . . .[23]

Mental illness and depression is another example requiring generalist multiskilled individual practitioners. Most of these illnesses are mild and caused by a somato-psycho-socio-semiotic mix of problems and have little 'biological aetiology' – the angst of modern society – compared to the major depressions. Not surprisingly then the most beneficial treatment for these is an ongoing personal therapeutic relationship over time rather than the use of medications.[24]

To the community at large, primary care offers significantly better access to needed care and provides that care more equitably by removing financial barriers. This is particularly so in disadvantaged and marginalised communities.

Important health gains can be achieved by focusing interventions on the health of the entire population (or significant subpopulations) as well as individuals. These interventions are a shared responsibility between public policies in areas outside the health system and health-centred policies from within. Aligning these policies would help to overcome important factors contributing to health inequalities, in particular the issues of absolute and relative income as well as the availability of social infrastructure and social capital, and enhance the fundamental tenet of equity in health, equity being

> . . . the absence of systematic and potentially remediable differences in one or more aspect of health across populations of population subgroups defined socially, economically, demographically, or geographically. (cited in reference 25)

WHERE IS THE PRIMARY (HEALTH) CARE MOVEMENT LEADING?

Firstly it needs to be acknowledged that there remain many confusions and misconceptions about what is meant by primary (health) care. Is primary care being set up to replace the arguably highly successful models of general practice/family medicine, which in the view of some are seen as failing? Or is primary care being set up as a panacea for the government's inability to control the expenditure of an increasingly technology-based disease model of health services? Can primary care fill the void where general practice/family medicine apparently has 'failed'?

Even though each government is challenged to make the system more responsive to patient needs, they are equally challenged to bring the health system components and their providers under financial control. Hence policy makers have – in recent years – accepted the importance of primary health care as a key strategy to further the achievement of these goals.[20] Nevertheless, they not infrequently contemplate, organise and implement reforms that are in direct contradiction to the primary healthcare goals.

While improved disease care, provided by multidisciplinary and multidimensional teams, is the cost-containment dream of governments and policy makers, the unforseen consequence of such a reform drive are steeply rising administrative costs.[26,27] There is no doubt that multidisciplinary care is needed to achieve all of the goals of primary care – yet teams are not required in many, if not most, situations. Where then would primary care teams most effectively and efficiently be located? Dawson proposed the concept of primary and secondary health centres with broader teams that could support GPs/family physicians in their practices by providing higher levels of specialised care and linkages to domiciliary services.

There is strong evidence about the effectiveness of well-functioning teams, for example for those with serious mental illness or complex and multisystem chronic disease, or the frail elderly, and for community development work in disadvantaged populations.[28] However, teams have been shown not to be a substitute of the *ongoing personal doctor–patient relationship.*

While doctor–nurse substitution may have the potential to reduce a doctor's workload and direct healthcare costs,[29,30] achieving such reductions depends on the particular context of care. A doctor's workload may well remain unchanged either because nurses are deployed to meet previously unmet patient need, or because nurses generate demand for care where previously there was none.[30] Cost savings also depend on the magnitude of the salary differential between doctors and nurses, and may easily be offset by the lower productivity of nurses compared to doctors.[29,30]

A concern, particularly for developing countries, is the pressure to accept as the only way of health system reform a market-oriented approach rather than the development of a primary healthcare model based on social justice and human rights principles.[31,32] Table 20.2 compares the different assumptions and key features of market and a social justice approaches.

TABLE 20.2 Neoliberal and social justice approaches to health: a comparison[32]

NEOLIBERAL APPROACH TO HEALTH	SOCIAL JUSTICE/HUMAN RIGHTS APPROACH TO HEALTH
Underlying assumptions	Alternative assumptions
1 Economic growth, within a globalised 'free' market is the aim	1 Fair distribution and sustainable use of resources is the aim
2 Health is what you get from a health service	2 Health is what you get from meeting basic rights
3 International aid, with conditionalities to enforce certain policies, is the only way to finance health	3 Sovereign states must provide for their people's rights without outside interference
4 Democracy is alive and well in the developed world and is the model for the developing world	4 Democracy is in crisis everywhere. Self-determination of nation states and a rules-based system of international governance are required
Key features	
• Addresses symptoms, short term	• Addresses root causes, long term
• Promotes 'silver (medical) bullets'	• Promotes the meeting of people's health rights
• Promotes interventions delivered through health services	• Promotes public works to free people from miserable living conditions
• Identifies charity and international aid as the only sources of funds for health	• Identifies income redistribution and economic justice as sources of funds for health
• Maintains the status quo of extreme concentrations of wealth and power	• Demands a fair and rational international economic order
• Focuses on individual behaviour and tends to blame victims	• Focuses on structural poverty and violence and finds the causes of them in the system

THE BENEFITS OF A GENERALIST-ORIENTED HEALTH SYSTEM

So how poorly are generalist primary care providers really doing? Or should the question rather be – how much better are generalist primary care providers doing for most common conditions in the community? The overwhelming answer is 'very well' indeed.

Barbara Starfield has examined the performance of primary care in great detail, showing the overwhelming benefits in terms of health and economic outcomes of healthcare environments with a generalist rather than specialist orientation.[3,25,33,34] Tables 20.3–20.5 detail the many benefits of primary care orientation on health outcomes and health service delivery.

It has been argued that specialists are better at dealing with their specific diseases.[35] However when comparing disease specific services, e.g. in diabetes or hypertension, no significant difference in outcomes were found.[36] Some studies that initially demonstrated benefits of specialist care were subsequently found to show no difference in outcomes when study design and sample size issues (case-mix bias and physician clustering) were appropriately taken into account.[37]

Comparisons become even more difficult given that most of the studies look at patients without co-morbidities and only describe disease-specific outcomes. However most patients encountered in primary care will have co-morbidities that makes it impossible to judge which mode of service delivery achieves overall better *personal health*, the indicator that matters most to our patients.[12,13,17]

Overall comparison studies of care processes and outcomes between different providers and different healthcare settings are problematic, and results have to be viewed with caution.[26] Nonetheless in global terms, primary care is by no means inferior to specialist-based care.[25]

TABLE 20.3 Impact of higher primary care provider supply on health outcomes (compiled from Starfield[3])

	COMMENTS
US	
Higher primary care to population ratio	
Lower all-cause mortality:	Controlled for sociodemographic measures (percentage of elderly, urban, and minorities; income; unemployment; pollution) and lifestyle factors (seatbelt use; obesity; smoking)
• heart disease	
• cancer	
• stroke	
Increased life span	
Lower infant mortality	
Lower low-birth weight	
Lower poor self-rated health	
Higher primary care ratio overcomes income inequality	
Increased life expectancy	Controlled for age, sex, race/ethnicity, education, paid work, hourly wage, family income, health insurance, physical health, smoking
Lower total mortality:	
• stroke mortality	
• post-neonatal mortality	
Higher specialist to primary care physician ratio	
Higher mortality	
Higher primary care physician ratio in non-urban counties	
2% lower all-cause mortality:	
• 4% lower heart disease mortality	
• 3% lower cancer mortality	
Higher family physician ratio compared with general internists and paediatricians	
Lower mortality	
• lower stroke mortality	
UK	
1 additional GP (15–20% increase) per 10 000 population is associated with a 6% drop in overall mortality	

TABLE 20.3 *cont*

Ratio of GPs to population is significantly associated with:	After controlling for socio-economic deprivation and partnership size, differences disappeared. The authors concluded that:
• all-cause mortality • mortality from acute MI • avoidable mortality • acute hospital admission for both acute and chronic conditions • teenage pregnancies	• the structural characteristics of primary care practices may have a greater impact on health outcomes than do the mere presence of primary care physicians

TABLE 20.4 Impact of patients' relationship with primary care providers and primary care facilities (compiled from Starfield[3])

	COMMENTS
US	
People identifying with a primary care physician are healthier	Regardless of their initial health or various demographic characteristics
Spain	
Introduced system that patients had to see a GP prior to seeing any other physician, areas that introduced the system first saw reduced mortality from hypertension and stroke	
Canada	
Better post-operative outcomes: • better for children who were referred to specialist for recurrent otitis media and tonsillitis than those who self-referred	Authors argue that specialist intervention was more appropriate for referred patients

TABLE 20.5 Presence of primary care attributes and achievement of healthcare services (compiled from Starfield[3])

	COMMENTS
US	
Services that have primary care attributes: • are up to date with screening • are up to date with immunisations • are up to date on health habit counselling • have less accident and emergency care	
Patients who receive care from service with primary care attributes: • 5% fewer report poor health • 6% fewer report depression	Of those reporting best primary care experience, 8% fewer reported poor health and 10% fewer reported depression
Brazil	
Patients who receive care from service with primary care attributes: • report better health	Difference remains after adjusting for age, chronic or recent illness, household wealth, educational level

SUMMARY POINTS

- The term 'primary care' was first suggested by Dawson in 1920 as part of the social health movement to address healthcare deficiencies and health inequalities. The concept was expanded, adopted and promulgated again in 1978 in the Alma-Ata Declaration.
- The Alma-Ata Declaration proposed a primary healthcare strategy that would overcome health inequalities and guarantee 'health for all' by integrating prevention and health promotion with curative and co-ordinated care for complicated disease at the point of first contact with the healthcare system.
- Primary healthcare service models were seen as an enhancement to the care provided by GPs/family physicians through improved organisational structures and the integration with or linkage to other health care providers.
- Shifting morbidity burdens require better integrated care to enhance the personal health experience, to improve disease-specific management and to contain costs.
- Care co-ordination is particularly needed at times of transition within the personal illness trajectory.
- Self-rated health is a powerful predictor of mortality, beyond prevailing disease models, yet healthcare providers may find their perception of a patient's health to significantly differ from the patient's view of their health.
- Effective primary care requires generalist multiskilled practitioners, not multiple single-skilled providers. Their effectiveness arises from an ongoing personal healing relationship based on knowledge and trust.
- It is not yet clear if policy makers see 'primary care' as a means to enhance the timely delivery of appropriate care to those in need or as a 'cost-containment' tool.
- There is overwhelming ecological evidence that generalist-orientated primary care systems achieve better health outcomes and are more cost-effective.

CHAPTER 21

The healthcare vortex: a metaphor for a sustainable healthcare system

The World will not evolve past its current state of crisis by using the same thinking that created the situation.

Albert Einstein

Ordinary words convey only what we know already; it is from metaphors that we can best get hold of something fresh.

Aristotle, Rhetoric 1410b[39]

By shifting focus to relationships instead of separate entities, scientists made an amazing discovery ... system properties are awesomely elegant in their simplicity and constancy throughout the universe, from suborganic to biological and ecological systems, and mental and social systems, as well.

Joanna Macy

Einstein, Aristotle and Macy all allude to the same necessity, to see things – in this case *health* and *health care* – in a different light. Since the preceding chapters have repeatedly indicated the intricate interdependent nature of health, illness and disease it makes common sense to adopt a complex adaptive systems framework as a way forward to understanding, redefining and reshaping health care.

Before proceeding let us recall the emerging patterns from the first four sections:
■ The historical origins of medicine live on into our times. Health and health care are social constructs; ill people are anxious and concerned and want to understand

their illness; the doctor, being part of the community knows and understands the subtleties of the community and he knows 'medicine'; and in the consultation patients share their illness experience with their trusted doctor as a means to regain their health (or achieve healing).

■ Inherent in modern society's sub/consciousness are three notions: 'illness' is a loss of balance; the 'mind–body split' drives medical sciences; and 'knowing' is a complex personal phenomenon. The historical primacy of the consultation remains the defining characteristic of medicine as a discipline.

■ Healing is the 'core value' of medicine which shapes the continuing and person-centred care process of the consultation. These values and processes remain the foundations for achieving the balance of somato-psycho-socio-semiotic health.

■ Societal values and structures directly and indirectly determine the health and life expectancy of individuals. Changing societal approaches to social determinants of health can be more beneficial to achieving better personal health than providing more healthcare services.

Complex adaptive systems are best understood through metaphors, metaphors are able to describe the multidimensional and interconnected phenomena of the real world that are otherwise not easily accessible to most people.

THE HEALTHCARE VORTEX

The *healthcare vortex* is a fitting metaphor to describe the layered and interconnected relationships between health, health care and the healthcare system, and as a result provides a mental framework for health systems reform (*see* Figure 21.1).

In health and health system terms the vortex metaphor describes the constant adaptation and adjustments to changing healthcare needs and healthcare priorities, technologies and economic considerations. The healthcare vortex has a focal point around which the patterns of the system stabilise; however, when the focal point is poorly articulated or understood, the system may become dysfunctional and unresponsive to societal needs. Pellegrino and Thomasma remind us that pseudo-values have influenced health care in our time:

> The process of modernization is associated with bureaucratization and technology, which have become values in themselves. They are prime shapers of the cognitive style of our culture and of modern medicine.[40]

PRIMARY CARE AND THE HEALTHCARE VORTEX

All systems are bound by their history. Social systems also self-organise around their core value(s). This book has traced both and shown that health and illness are primarily constructed in personal and experiential terms, and that medical care promotes *health* through a healing doctor–patient relationship. Regaining *health* means finding meaning in or making sense out of the illness experiences. The somato-psycho-socio-semiotic model of *health* and *illness* articulates this process.

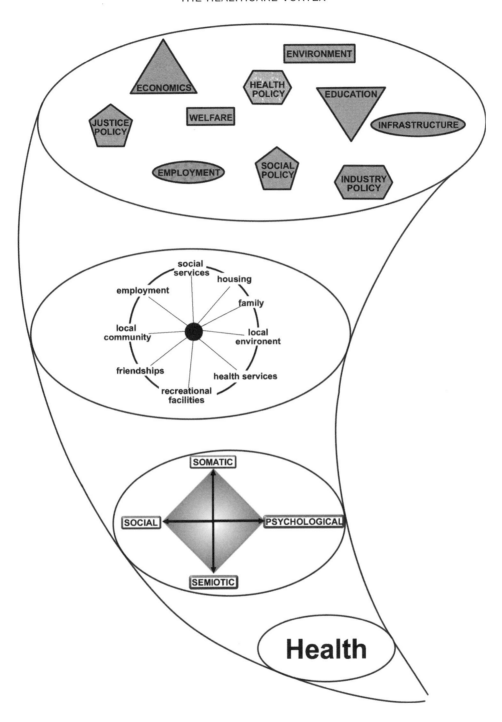

Figure 21.1 The healthcare vortex.

Achieving best possible *personal health* – as shown in Sections 3 and 4 – is dependent on numerous interconnected factors, many of which are not yet taken fully into account by health service planners and policy makers (*see* Figure 21.1). In fact the physician healers' role in general practice/family medicine has been increasingly devalued by the push of an industrial model of primary care.[41]

The success of the health system must be measured against its core value – improving *personal health*. Since systems achieve what they are designed to do, the design and the implementation of the health system must constantly reflect back on the core value – improving *personal health*. And since there are many external factors impacting on the patterns, structure and processes of the health system, their influences must also be assessed against the core value – how do they impact on *personal health*? Feedback loops are the mode by which systems adjust, and thus feedback allows the fine-tuning of the health system around its core value – improving *personal health*.

SIMPLE RULES DRIVE THE HEALTHCARE VORTEX

The foundations of *personal health*, i.e. the understanding of the nature of health, illness and healing, must remain central to the structure and processes of the health system. They include the notions of:

- *person-centred care*
- the therapeutic relationship requiring a *predominant continuing relationship with a personal physician*
- healing means *making sense* out of the illness experience, rather than *per se* the 'cure' of a 'disease'.

Those who truly want to achieve an effective healthcare system will do their utmost to adhere to these basic rules. In fact it is *simple rules* that drive complex adaptive systems effectively.

IMPLICATIONS FOR PRIMARY CARE

The healthcare vortex is an important metaphor for the activities of the health system and the design of healthcare policies.

The core characteristics of general practice/family medicine – accessibility, continuity of care, sufficient time in the consultation and the doctor–patient relationship – provide a solid foundation for the emerging primary care system. Studies have confirmed the positive relationships between the attributes of general practice/family medicine and the outcomes of care – satisfaction, self-rated health and cost.

Patient satisfaction is associated with accessibility, continuity of care, consultation length and the doctor–patient relationship. Improvement in patient health is related to continuity of care, consultation length, doctor–patient relationship and the implementation of preventive activities. And continuity of care, consultation length, doctor–patient communication and preventive care are associated with lower healthcare costs. However, co-ordination of care shows only a weak associations with health outcomes.[41]

WHAT SHOULD BE THE 'CORE VALUE' OF PRIMARY CARE

We have provided compelling evidence that medicine's core value should remain as improving *personal health*, though not everyone will agree with us. At a time of exponentially rising healthcare costs, the argument of reforms needing to achieve cost containment sounds convincing, superficially. However, we believe that many of the costs are costs incurred through policy decisions in other domains that have been shown to have a substantial negative impact on patients' health.

THE PLACE OF PRIMARY CARE TEAMS

Dawson in his early models of primary and secondary health centres did not see the roles of the broader primary care teams as substituting for the GP *but collaborating around care of the individual, in their home and local community contexts.*

> We begin with the home, and the services, preventive and curative, which revolve round it, viz., those of the doctor, dentist, pharmacist, nurse, midwife, and health visitor. These we style domiciliary services, and they constitute the periphery of the scheme, the remainder of which is mainly institutional in character. A Health Centre is an institution wherein are brought together various medical services, preventive and curative, so as to form one organisation. Health Centres may be either Primary or Secondary, the former denoting a more simple, and the latter a more specialised service.[7]

Nevertheless the current primary care reform agendas strongly focus on the idea of substituting GP/family physician care for care by nurses. We alluded to the flaws in this concept, and again point out that what makes medical care effective and efficient – both in achieving improved health and containing costs – is based on the *person-centred ongoing therapeutic doctor–patient relationship.* As far back as 1978 McWhinney voiced his concerns about the detrimental consequences of these emerging developments:

> If it is proposed that a craft skill be mechanized, we must examine very closely the full consequences of this act. These must include the consequences for the physician–patient relationship, the consequences for the physician's feeling for his task, and the long-term consequences for the patient and his family'.[42]

THE PRIMARY CARE REFORM AGENDA

Experience tells us that reform often leads to undesired outcomes, dismantling the very best parts of the old without gaining corresponding benefits from the new. Thus the question arises: '*Is there common ground from which to explore the space of possibilities for effective and efficient health services?*'.

One aspect not taken sufficient account of is the consequences of 'the many non-health policy decisions' – e.g. limited access to education or economic policies that threaten workplace security – that impact on *personal health* and thereby negatively impact on health service demands. This must become a priority concern to all governments when deciding on any new policy initiative.

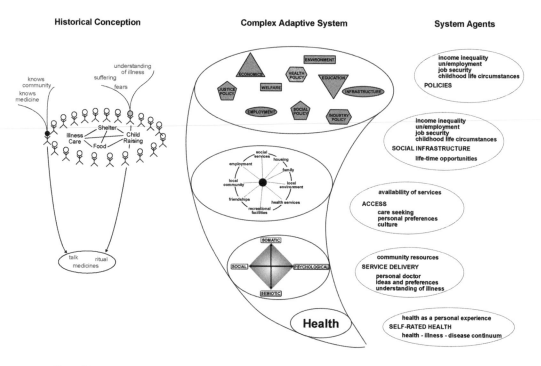

Figure 21.2 The healthcare vortex in context.

We are not the first and won't be the last, to highlight the *proven strength of personal doctoring* as a core element that needs to be preserved in the ongoing reforms of primary care. Steinar Westin remarked:

> In a world plagued with unforeseen discontinuities, general practice will need to maintain its core of 'personal doctoring'. Meeting people at the primary care level provides unique opportunities of being sensitive and responsive also to unexpected changes in society, and in some areas even making contributions to the directions of change[43]

and David Thom summarises the evidence as follows:

> The physician–patient relationship is recognized as having an essential role in the process of medical care, providing the context in which caring and healing can occur. Patient trust in the physician has been proposed as a key feature of this relationship. There are several potential benefits to patient trust, including increased satisfaction, adherence to treatment, and continuity of care. Trust may also be associated with lower transaction costs, such as those incurred by a need to reassure patients (e.g. ordering additional tests and referrals) or by inefficiencies due to incomplete disclosure of information by the patient.[44]

Figure 21.2 shows the translation of the historical concepts of health, health service and healthcare needs into the complex adaptive system concept of the healthcare vortex, and reiterates some of the important system agents for each of the different levels within the vortex. Our needs and our expectations as mortal beings have remained unchanged over the centuries, despite the enormous growth in societal, scientific and technological advancements. The future of medicine, and in particular the future of primary care, is its ability to adapt to the changing expressions of the otherwise unchanging societal expectations of improvement in the *personal health experience*. This latter point needs to be re-appreciated by patients, doctors and healthcare planners alike.

CONCLUSIONS

Primary health care has the capacity to improve the health of individuals and communities. The potential arises from its ability to provide personalised responses to individual needs, and community-based responses to adverse factors impacting on health and the health experience.

The potential benefits of primary health care will only be achieved if the health system develops a clear vision and goals. Having a clear vision and goals will enable health planners to assess the impact of all societal activity on health, and thus will foster the development of appropriate political, organisational and resource responses.

These are most likely to emerge by embracing a complex adaptive system framework – metaphorically described here as the *healthcare vortex* – that recognises the importance of the various perspectives on health and health care, encompassing history, philosophy, sociology, biology, life sciences and organisational studies, as well as reductionist sciences where appropriate.

The simplistic approaches of the past – which failed to recognise the dynamic, interconnected and participatory dimensions of complex adaptive systems – have had limited success in improving health and health care, and have led to many negative unintended outcomes that in fact compounded the prevailing problem.

A complexity approach provides new ways of understanding health, health care and the healthcare system. General practice/family medicine should take the lead in the unfolding history and philosophy of primary (health) care, confident in the knowledge of their ability to achieve improved health based on their well-tested approach of an *ongoing person-centred therapeutic doctor–patient relationship*.

SUMMARY POINTS

- Achieving the best possible *personal health* is dependent on numerous interconnected factors all of which must be fully taken into account by health service planners and policy makers.
- The success of the health system must be measured against its core value, improved *personal health*.
- The foundations of *personal health*, i.e. the understanding of the nature of health, illness and healing, must remain central to the structure and processes of the health system and include three conceptual elements
  — person-centred care
  — a continuing relationship with a personal physician
  — healing as a sense-making process.
- The proven strength of personal doctoring needs to be preserved in the ongoing reforms of primary care.
- The future of medicine, and in particular the future of primary care, is its ability to adapt to the changing expressions of the otherwise unchanging societal expectations of improvement in the *personal health experience*.

REFERENCES

1 Dostoevsky F. *The Brothers Karamazov*. New York: Farrar, Straus and Giroux, 2002.
2 Ackoff R. The future of operations research is past. *Journal of the Operational Research Society*. 1979; **30**(2): 93–104.
3 Starfield B, Shi L and Macinko J. Contribution of primary care to health systems and health. *Milbank Quarterly*. 2005; **83**: 457–502.
4 Gask L. Powerlessness, control, and complexity: the experience of family physicians in a group model HMO. *Annals of Family Medicine*. 2004; **2**: 150–5.
5 Green L, Fryer G, Yawn B, Lanier D and Dovey S. The ecology of medical care revisited. *New England Journal of Medicine*. 2001; **344**: 2021–5.
6 World Health Organization. *Declaration of Alma-Ata*. International Conference on Primary Health Care, 6–12 September 1978, Alma-Ata, USSR. Geneva: World Health Organization, 1978.
7 Lord Dawson. *Interim Report on the Future Provisions of Medical and Allied Services*. London: United Kingdom Ministry of Health. Consultative Council on Medical Allied Services, HMSO, 1920.
8 Kelleher H. Why primary health care offers a more comprehensive approach to tackling health inequalities than primary care. *Australian Journal of Primary Health Care*. 2001; **7**: 57–61.
9 Pan American Health Organization, World Health Organization. *Regional Declaration on the New Orientations for Primary Health Care* (Declaration of Montevideo) 2005. www.paho.org/English/GOV/CD/cd46-decl-e.pdf (accessed 6 July 2006).
10 Murray C and Lopez AE. *The Global Burden of Disease*. Geneva: World Health Organization, Harvard School of Public Health, World Bank, 1996.

11 Lynn J and Adamson D. *Living Well at the End of Life. Adapting health care to serious chronic illness in old age.* Santa Monica, CA: Rand Health, 2003.

12 Martin C and Rohan B. Chronic illness care as a balancing act. A qualitative study. *Australian Family Physician.* 2002; **31**: 55–9.

13 Muir Gray J. *The Resourceful Patient – 21st Century health care.* Online book, 2003. www. resourcefulpatient.org/text/text.htm (accessed 6 July 2006).

14 Martin C, Robinson R and Peterson C. *The Care of Chronic Illness in General Practice. Focus groups with chronic disease self help groups: report to the Family Medicine Research Foundation,* Melbourne: RACGP, 2003.

15 Wagner E and Groves T. Care for chronic diseases. The efficacy of coordinated and patient centred care is established, but now is the time to test its effectiveness. *British Medical Journal.* 2002; **325**: 913–14.

16 Martin C. *The Care of Chronic Illness in General Practice.* Canberra: PhD Thesis Australian National University, 1999.

17 Lara-Muñoz C and Feinstein A. How should quality of life be measured? *Journal of Investigative Medicine.* 1999; **47**: 17–24.

18 Idler E and Benyamini Y. Self-rated health and mortality: a review of twenty-seven community studies. *Journal of Health and Social Behaviour.* 1997; **38**: 21–37.

19 Tarimo E and Webster EG. *Primary Health Care Concepts and Challenges in a Changing World: Alma-Ata revisited.* Current Concerns SHS Paper number 7, WHO/SHS/CC/94.2. Geneva: World Health Organization, 1994.

20 Kekki P. *Primary Health Care and the Millennium Development Goals: issues for discussion.* Madrid: World Health Organization. The Global Meeting on Future Strategic Directions for Primary Health Care, 27–29 October 2003. www.who.int/entity/chronic_conditions/ primary_health_care/en/mdgs_final.pdf (accessed 6 July 2006).

21 Maynard A and Bloor K. Primary care and health care reform: the need to reflect before reforming. *Health Policy.* 1995; **31**: 171–81.

22 Maynard A and Bloor K. Universal coverage and cost control: the United Kingdom National Health Service. *Journal of Health and Human Services Administration.* 1998; **20**: 423–41.

23 Maynard A. Is high technology medicine cost effective? *Physics in Medicine and Biology.* 1989; **34**: 407–18.

24 Kayita J. *Palliative Care in Resource-Constrained Settings for People Living with HIV and Other Life-Threatening Illnesses: lessons learned from Uganda.* http://hab.hrsa.gov/publications/ palliative/palliative_care_uganda.htm (accessed 6 July 2006).

25 Ellis P and Smith D. Treating depression: the beyond blue guidelines for treating depression in primary care 'Not so much what you do but that you keep doing it'. *Medical Journal of Australia.* 2002; **176** (Suppl): S77–S83.

26 Starfield B, Shi L, Grover A and Macinko J. The effects of specialist supply on populations' health: assessing the evidence. *Health Affairs – Web Exclusive.* 2005; **W5**: 97–105.

27 Giuffrida A, Gravelle H and Roland M. Measuring quality of care with routine data: avoiding confusion between performance indicators and health outcomes. *British Medical Journal.* 1999; **319**: 94–8.

28 Giuffrida A, Gravelle H and Sutton M. Efficiency and administrative costs in primary care. *Journal of Health Economics.* 2000; **19**: 983–1006.

29 Bower P, Campbell S, Bojke C and Sibbald B. Team structure, team climate and the quality of care in primary care: an observational study. *Quality and Safety in Health Care*. 2003; **12**: 273–9.

30 Laurant MGH, Hermens RPMG, Braspenning JCC, Sibbald B and Grol RPTM. Impact of nurse practitioners on workload of general practitioners: randomised controlled trial. *British Medical Journal*. 2004; **328**: 927–32.

31 Laurant M, Reeves D, Hermens R *et al*. Substitution of doctors by nurses in primary care (Cochrane review). *The Cochrane Library, Issue 2*. Oxford: Update Software, 2005.

32 Jensen B, Schnack K and Simovska V. *Critical Environmental and Health Education Research Issues and Challenges*. Copenhagen: Research Centre for Environmental and Health Education, The Danish University of Education, 2000. www.rec.hu/seminar6/doc/AC_Social_Capital.doc (accessed 6 July 2006).

33 *Neoliberal Ideology in the World Health Organization: effects on global public health policy and practice*. http://lists.kabissa.org/lists/archives/public/pha-exchange/msg01808.html (accessed 6 July 2006).

34 Starfield B. *Primary Care. Balancing Health Needs, Services, and Technology* (revised edition). New York, Oxford: Oxford University Press, 1998.

35 Phillips RJ, Dodoo M and Green L. Adding more specialists is not likely to improve population health: is anybody listening? *Health Affairs – Web Exclusive*. 2005; **W5**: 111–14.

36 Harrold L, Field T and Gurwitz J. Knowledge, patterns of care, and outcomes of care for generalists and specialists. *Journal of General Internal Medicine*. 1999; **14**: 499–511.

37 Greenfield S, Rogers W, Mangotich M, Carney M and Tarlov A. Outcomes of patients with hypertension and non-insulin-dependent diabetes mellitus treated by different systems and specialties. *Journal of the American Medical Association*. 1995; **274**: 1436–44.

38 Greenfield S, Kaplan S, Kahn R, Ninomiya J and Griffith J. Profiling care provided by different groups of physicians: effects of patient case-mix (bias) and physician-level clustering on quality assessment results. *Annals of Internal Medicine*, 2002; **136**: 111–21.

39 Aristotle. *Rhetoric*. www.public.iastate.edu/~honeyl/Rhetoric/index.html (accessed 6 July 2006).

40 Pellegrino E and Thomasma D. *A Philosophical Basis of Medical Practice. Towards a philosophy and ethic of the healing professions*. New York Oxford: Oxford University Press, 1981.

41 Iliffe S. From general practice to primary care: the industrialisation of family medicine in Britain. *Journal of Public Health Policy*. 2002; **23**: 33–43.

42 Sans-Corrales M, Pujol-Ribera E, Gene-Badia J *et al*. Family medicine attributes related to satisfaction, health and costs. *Family Practice* 2006: **23**: 308–16.

43 McWhinney I. Medical knowledge and the rise of technology. *Journal of Medical Philosophy*. 1978; **3**: 293–304.

44 Westin S. The market is a strange creature: family medicine meeting the challenges of the changing political and socioeconomic structure. *Family Practice*. 1995; **12**: 394–401.

45 Thom D and Stanford Trust Study Physicians. Physician behaviors that predict patient trust. *Journal of Family Practice*. 2001; **50**: 323–8.

Appendix: Declaration of Alma-Ata

INTERNATIONAL CONFERENCE ON PRIMARY HEALTH CARE, 6–12 SEPTEMBER 1978, ALMA-ATA, USSR

The International Conference on Primary Health Care, meeting in Alma-Ata this twelfth day of September in the year nineteen hundred and seventy-eight, expressing the need for urgent action by all governments, all health and development workers, and the world community to protect and promote the health of all the people of the world, hereby makes the following

DECLARATION:

I

The Conference strongly reaffirms that health, which is a state of complete physical, mental and social wellbeing, and not merely the absence of disease or infirmity, is a fundamental human right and that the attainment of the highest possible level of health is a most important world-wide social goal whose realization requires the action of many other social and economic sectors in addition to the health sector.

II

The existing gross inequality in the health status of the people particularly between developed and developing countries as well as within countries is politically, socially and economically unacceptable and is, therefore, of common concern to all countries.

III

Economic and social development, based on a New International Economic Order, is of basic importance to the fullest attainment of health for all and to the reduction of the gap between the health status of the developing and developed countries. The promotion and protection of the health of the people is essential to sustained economic and social development and contributes to a better quality of life and to world peace.

IV

The people have the right and duty to participate individually and collectively in the planning and implementation of their health care.

V

Governments have a responsibility for the health of their people which can be fulfilled only by the provision of adequate health and social measures. A main social target of governments, international organizations and the whole world community in the coming decades should be the attainment by all peoples of the world by the year 2000 of a level of health that will permit them to lead a socially and economically productive life. Primary health care is the key to attaining this target as part of development in the spirit of social justice.

VI

Primary health care is essential health care based on practical, scientifically sound and socially acceptable methods and technology made universally accessible to individuals and families in the community through their full participation and at a cost that the community and country can afford to maintain at every stage of their development in the spirit of self-reliance and self-determination. It forms an integral part both of the country's health system, of which it is the central function and main focus, and of the overall social and economic development of the community. It is the first level of contact of individuals, the family and community with the national health system bringing health care as close as possible to where people live and work, and constitutes the first element of a continuing health care process.

VII

Primary health care:
1 reflects and evolves from the economic conditions and sociocultural and political characteristics of the country and its communities and is based on the application of the relevant results of social, biomedical and health services research and public health experience;
2 addresses the main health problems in the community, providing promotive, preventive, curative and rehabilitative services accordingly;
3 includes at least: education concerning prevailing health problems and the methods of preventing and controlling them; promotion of food supply and proper nutrition; an adequate supply of safe water and basic sanitation; maternal and child health care, including family planning; immunization against the major infectious diseases; prevention and control of locally endemic diseases; appropriate treatment of common diseases and injuries; and provision of essential drugs;

4   involves, in addition to the health sector, all related sectors and aspects of national and community development, in particular agriculture, animal husbandry, food, industry, education, housing, public works, communications and other sectors; and demands the coordinated efforts of all those sectors;

5   requires and promotes maximum community and individual self-reliance and participation in the planning, organization, operation and control of primary health care, making fullest use of local, national and other available resources; and to this end develops through appropriate education the ability of communities to participate;

6   should be sustained by integrated, functional and mutually supportive referral systems, leading to the progressive improvement of comprehensive health care for all, and giving priority to those most in need;

7   relies, at local and referral levels, on health workers, including physicians, nurses, midwives, auxiliaries and community workers as applicable, as well as traditional practitioners as needed, suitably trained socially and technically to work as a health team and to respond to the expressed health needs of the community.

VIII

All governments should formulate national policies, strategies and plans of action to launch and sustain primary health care as part of a comprehensive national health system and in coordination with other sectors. To this end, it will be necessary to exercise political will, to mobilize the country's resources and to use available external resources rationally.

IX

All countries should cooperate in a spirit of partnership and service to ensure primary health care for all people since the attainment of health by people in any one country directly concerns and benefits every other country. In this context the joint WHO/ UNICEF report on primary health care constitutes a solid basis for the further development and operation of primary health care throughout the world.

X

An acceptable level of health for all the people of the world by the year 2000 can be attained through a fuller and better use of the world's resources, a considerable part of which is now spent on armaments and military conflicts. A genuine policy of independence, peace, détente and disarmament could and should release additional resources that could well be devoted to peaceful aims and in particular to the acceleration of social and economic development of which primary health care, as an essential part, should be allotted its proper share.

The International Conference on Primary Health Care calls for urgent and effective national and international action to develop and implement primary health care throughout the world and particularly in developing countries in a spirit of technical cooperation and in keeping with a New International Economic Order. It urges governments, WHO and UNICEF, and other international organizations, as well as multilateral and bilateral agencies, nongovernmental organizations, funding agencies, all health workers and the whole world community to support national and international commitment to primary health care and to channel increased technical and financial support to it, particularly in developing countries.

The Conference calls on all the aforementioned to collaborate in introducing, developing and maintaining primary health care in accordance with the spirit and content of this Declaration.

Index

Page numbers in italic refer to tables or figures.

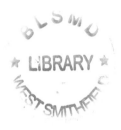